# Nonsurgical Peri-orbital Rejuvenation

Shoib A. Myint
Editor

# Nonsurgical Peri-orbital Rejuvenation

Springer

*Editor*
Shoib A. Myint, D.O., F.A.A.C.S., F.A.O.C.O.
Myint Facial Plastic & Cosmetic Surgery
University Medical Center
Valley Hospital
Las Vegas, NV, USA

Supplementary material for this volume can be accessed at http://springerimages.com/Videos/978-1-4614-8387-8.

ISBN 978-1-4614-8387-8 ISBN 978-1-4614-8388-5 (eBook)
DOI 10.1007/978-1-4614-8388-5
Springer New York Heidelberg Dordrecht London

Library of Congress Control Number: 2013947922



Printed on acid-free paper

Springer is part of Springer Science+Business Media (www.springer.com)

*In Loving Memory of R. Than Myint M.D.*
*This book is dedicated to Dahlia and Sophie.*

# Foreword

To be invited to write the Foreword to a text produced by a colleague is an honor and privilege in and of itself. To be invited by a former student is a special source of pride.

We have known Shoib Myint for more than 20 years. He was our student, resident, Fellow, and partner. After being in practice together for more than 10 years, his departure left not only a professional but also a personal void.

This new text, *Nonsurgical Peri-orbital Rejuvenation*, is the culmination of many years of collaborative efforts to fulfill a desire to continue to teach and write. The hope is to impart knowledge from experts so that practitioners can achieve outstanding results.

The use of Fillers and Injectibles as well as other nonsurgical modalities of treatment such as laser, radiofrequency energy, and peels represents a rapidly expanding group of procedures that are quickly becoming the forefront of cosmetic treatments. The text is enhanced with a section on anatomy and accompanying videos to aid in mastering the use of the procedures contained herein.

We are sure that this book will find its place in the library of all those who are in the field of cosmetic surgery.

Southfield, MI, USA

Frank Nesi
Geoffrey Gladstone

# Preface

This book is a result of the tremendous paradigm shift taking place in plastic surgery towards nonsurgical modalities in facial rejuvenation. I have witnessed this evolution accelerate over the last 5 years due to the increasing demand from patients desiring less downtime and faster recovery. I strongly feel that we have only begun to scratch the surface of what the future holds in less invasive techniques for not only the face but also the rest of the body.

The goal for this book is to offer the readers a platform of simple nonsurgical rejuvenating procedures with accompanying videos. It is catered for those beginning and intermediate surgeons who want to master the skills necessary to perform the following treatments.

This book would not have been possible without the dedication of the contributing authors who are leaders and innovators in their respective fields. I am grateful for their expertise and willingness to share their knowledge in the field of facial aesthetic surgery.

Finally I am grateful to my trainers, Frank Nesi and Geoff Gladstone, for sharing their friendship, patience, knowledge, and creativity. Above all, thank you both for giving me the gift of surgical artistry.

Las Vegas, NV, USA Shoib A. Myint, D.O.

# Contents

# Contributors

**John P. Arkins, B.S.** DeNova Research, Chicago, IL, USA

**Mark Berman, M.D., F.A.C.S.** Facial Plastic Surgery, University of Southern California, Los Angeles, CA, USA

**Tara E. Brennan, M.D.** Department of Otolaryngology – Head and Neck Surgery, University of Illinois at Chicago, Chicago, IL, USA

**Cat Nguyen Burkat, M.D., F.A.C.S.** University of Wisconsin School of Medicine and Public Health, Madison, WI, USA

**Steven H. Dayan, M.D., F.A.C.S.** Chicago Center for Facial Plastic Surgery, Chicago, IL, USA

DeNova Research, Chicago, IL, USA

Department of Otolaryngology-Head and Neck Surgery, University of Illinois at Chicago, Chicago, IL, USA

School of New Learning, DePaul University, Chicago, IL, USA

**Julie A. Edween, D.O., F.A.O.C.O., F.A.C.S.** Facial Plastic & Cosmetic Surgery, Beverly Hills, CA, USA

**Shubhra Goel, M.D., D.N.B.** Department of Ophthalmic Facial Plastic Surgery and Aesthetics, University of Wisconsin, Madison, WI, USA

**Megan C. Jack, M.D.** Sanctuary Medical Aesthetic Center, Boca Raton, FL, USA

**Bradley N. Lemke, M.D., F.A.C.S.** Lemke Facial Plastic and Cosmetic Surgery, Madison, WI, USA

**Corey S. Maas, M.D., F.A.C.S.** The Maas Clinic, University of California, San Francisco, San Francisco, CA, USA

**Jason N. Pozner, M.D.** Sanctuary Medical Aesthetic Center, Boca Raton, FL, USA

**Daniel I. Schlessinger** Northwestern University School of Medicine, Chicago, IL, USA

**Joel Schlessinger, M.D.** Director, Advanced Skin Research Center, Omaha, NE, USA

**Heidi A. Waldorf, M.D.** Director, Laser & Cosmetic Dermatology, Mount Sinai Medical Center, and Associate Clinical Professor Icahn School of Medicine, New York, NY, USA

Waldorf Dermatology & Laser Associates, PC, Nanuet, NY, USA

# Practical Anatomy of the Face and Eyelids: Cosmetic Applications

1

Shubhra Goel, Cat Nguyen Burkat, and Bradley N. Lemke

## Introduction

The evolving shift towards less invasive procedures for aesthetic facial rejuvenation naturally demands a more sophisticated understanding of facial anatomy. The outcome of any surgical or nonsurgical procedure can be optimized with a detailed understanding of the anatomical framework. An artistic and logical appreciation of the anatomical facial structures and their morphological variations is important in choosing and performing any procedure. This chapter highlights the practical anatomy of the upper and midface relevant to oculofacial cosmetic surgery.

S. Goel, M.D., D.N.B.
Department of Ophthalmic Facial Plastic Surgery and Aesthetics, University of Wisconsin, Madison, WI, USA

C.N. Burkat, M.D., F.A.C.S.
University of Wisconsin School of Medicine and Public Health, 2880 University Ave, Madison, WI 53705, USA

B.N. Lemke, M.D., F.A.C.S. (✉)
Lemke Facial Plastic and Cosmetic Surgery, Madison, WI, USA
e-mail: lemke@lemkefacialsurgery.com

## Facial Topography and Proportions

Facial proportions and topography may vary with age, gender, and ethnicity. It is essential to understand the standard basics of these proportions as well as their impact when considering any surgical or nonsurgical cosmetic procedure.

The normal human face extends vertically from the anterior hairline to the chin and is delineated laterally by the auricles. The inferior border of the face, also known as the jaw, is defined by the menton in the midline and the borders of the mandible laterally [1].

The shape and prominence of the forehead between the hairline and eyebrows is dependent on the frontal bone framework and the overlying subcutaneous tissue and muscle complex. The glabella is bordered on either side by the eyebrows, which run in an arched manner over the supraorbital rims. The periorbital region is divided into medial and lateral canthal areas and superior and inferior eyelid portions. The cheek lies over the prominent zygomatic bone to contribute to the youthfulness of the face. The cheek convexes anteriorly to merge with the lower lid to form the smooth eyelid-cheek junction. The cheek area is defined anteriorly by the external nose, nasolabial and labiomarginal folds, posteriorly by the anterior margin of the masseter muscle, superiorly by the infraorbital margin, and inferiorly by the mandible. The ideal location of the malar prominence is approximately 10 mm lateral and 15 mm inferior to the lateral

S.A. Myint (ed.), *Nonsurgical Peri-orbital Rejuvenation*, DOI 10.1007/978-1-4614-8388-5_1,

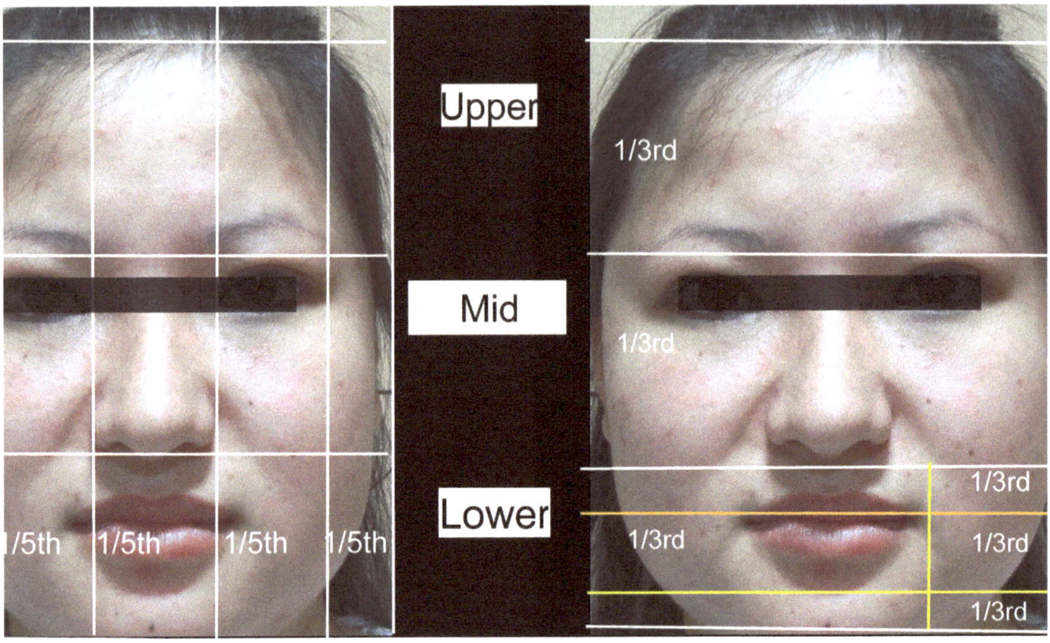


**Fig. 1.1** Dimensions of the ideal face divided into horizontal facial thirds and vertical fifths

canthal angle. Below the malar prominence lies the submalar triangle which is an inverted depressed triangular area of the middle third of the face, delineated superiorly by the zygomatic prominence, medially by the nasolabial fold, and laterally by the masseter muscle [1].

The ideal face has been described as five eye widths wide and eight eye widths high, and the normal location and dimensions of important structures are important to understand [2] (Fig. 1.1). Beauty has also been defined by the golden ratio (1.1.618) described as far as 300 BC, represented by the symbol pi [3]. The golden ratio is believed to be present in all animate and inanimate objects of nature and is defined as *when a line is divided into two unequal segments, the ratio of the longer segment to the whole line is equal to the ratio of the shorter segment to the longer one* (Fig. 1.2). Faces generally perceived to be beautiful have been intimately related to the golden ratio [4, 5]. For instance, the width of the mouth is pi times the width of the nose. This concept has been used to develop a "facial golden mask" that represents the ideal facial structures [6, 7].

## Facial Skin

The skin and the subcutaneous tissue over the face has been broadly classified into periorifacial and cervicofacial skin. The periorifacial skin around the eyes, nose, and mouth is thinnest on the face and has little or negligible subcutaneous fat. The muscle fibers in these areas are firmly adherent to the dermis of the skin and therefore clinically manifest as expression lines.

In contrast, the forehead, cheek, and neck are covered with thick skin with abundant subcutaneous fibrofatty tissue. The superficial musculoaponeurotic system (SMAS) is an example of this thicker cervicofacial tissue. Due to the presence of this thicker skin and subcutaneous tissue layer, these cervicofacial regions are less vulnerable to fine lines and wrinkle formation. The subcutaneous tissue and fat in these areas also define the facial framework and topography by softening bony prominences and filling in natural facial contours [8].

The skin in general is composed of the epidermis, dermis, and loose connective tissue with fat.

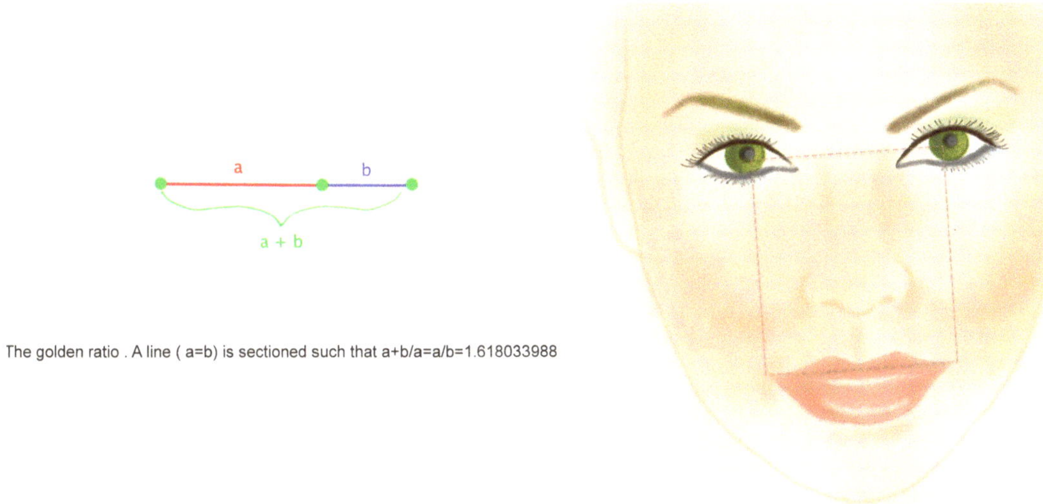


**Fig. 1.2** The golden ratio and beauty defined following the golden rule: The distance between the oral commissures when smiling should ideally be equal to the interpupillary distance and form a square

The outermost layer, the epidermis, is composed of four distinct layers—(1) keratinized and impermeable stratum corneum, (2) stratum granulosum, (3) vascular stratum spinosum, and (4) the cellular stratum basal (keratinocytes, melanocytes, fibroblasts) [7]. Although there is great variability in the thickness of the epidermis based on the particular anatomical site, it is on average 100 μm deep. The epidermis receives its nutrition from the highly vascular papillary dermis. Keratinocytes, which are the major cells of the epidermis, contribute to the genetic skin color of the epidermis. Keratin is the major protein that reacts with chemical peel agents, such as trichloroacetic acid (TCA) and phenol, to precipitate and form frost. $CO_2$ laser resurfacing evaporates the epidermis and a portion of dermis using water as a chromophore. If the epidermis and dermis are well hydrated, the results of laser resurfacing are therefore more uniform. Keratinocytes are sensitive to ultraviolet light exposure, which can cause structural damage to their DNA, leading to mutated precancerous cells [9].

The underlying dermis consists mainly of collagen and some elastic fibers (5 %). Approximately 500–1,000 μm thick, the dermis provides structural support to the epidermis and determines the thickness and elasticity of the skin. Dermal regeneration of the epidermis with any form of treatment like dermabrasion, laser resurfacing, or chemical peels depends on the integrity and function of the adnexal structures of the dermis. The dermis is subdivided into the superficial loose vascular layer of connective tissue called the papillary dermis and the deeper reticular layer rich in collagen and elastic fibers. To optimally correct wrinkles and scars with skin rejuvenation procedures, the dermal layer needs to be targeted to the appropriate depth based on the structure to be treated. Vascular lesions like port wine stains and telangiectasis are mainly dermal and can be minimized with dermal treatments. The dermis layer is compact, highly vascular, and also rich in nerve endings. Therefore, penetration of a needle into the dermal layer may meet resistance, be painful, and may cause superficial bruising.

The subcutaneous layer located beneath the dermal layer comprises primarily lobules of fatty tissue. Its thickness and presence of fascial connections are vital to the youthful face and are later important for volumetric analysis in the aging face.

The subcutaneous layer also functions as a buffer for skin trauma, as areas with abundant

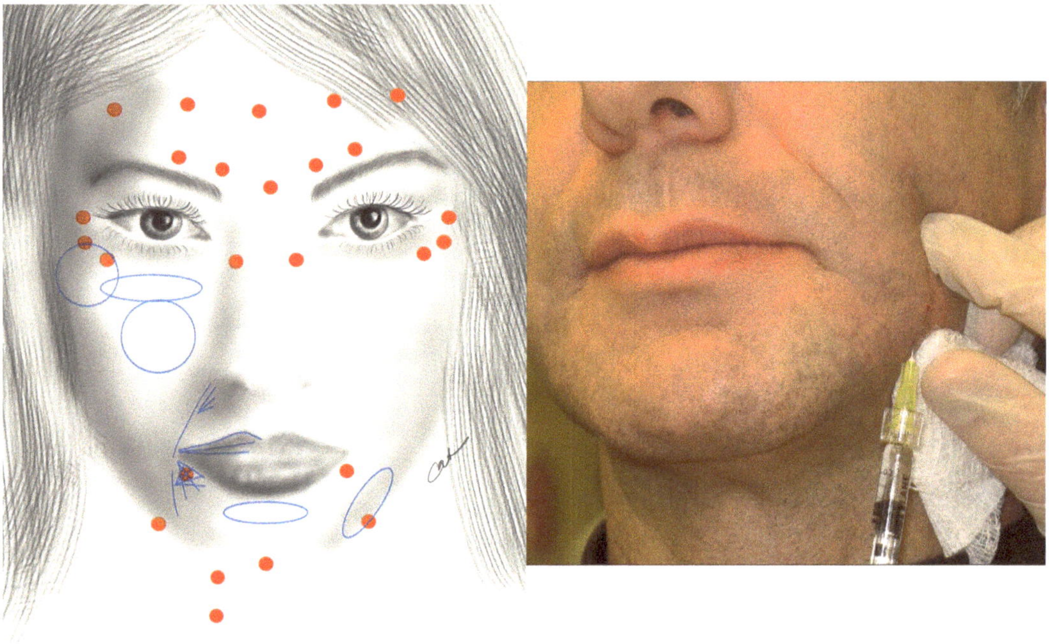

**Fig. 1.3** Common sites for facial botox (*red*) and dermal filler (*blue*) injections, based on underlying anatomy

subcutaneous tissue often heal faster and with less scaring than areas with thin or no subcutaneous tissue. Therefore, deep dermal penetration in areas of the face with almost no subcutaneous tissue, such as the lips, jawline, and neck, should be carefully approached. Dermal thickness in the nasolabial fold is approximately 1.32–1.55 mm. The diameter of the needle used to inject dermal fillers ranges between 0.3 and 0.4 mm with the length of the bevel being approximately 0.75–0.95 mm [10, 11]. Although the technique of using different angles for introduction of the needle into the superficial, mid, or deep dermis is still recommended, these variations with millimetric precision should be observed. The epidermal and dermal layers are thicker in the forehead area than the lower part of the face; thus, large volumes of fillers in the forehead area do not typically yield satisfactory results. In the temporal region where the skin is thin with visible superficial temporal vessels, meticulous injection of dermal fillers with delicate massage may avoid the Tyndall effect (Fig. 1.3) [12, 13].

## Facial Musculature and Soft Tissues

The face comprises the forehead, eyebrows, eyelids, cheek, and lower face subunits that are all closely interrelated. The face is enveloped by the superficial musculoaponeurotic system (SMAS), first described by Mitz and Peyronie [14]. The SMAS is a fibrous fascial tissue, extending from the temporalis and frontalis muscles superiorly to the platysma inferiorly, that interconnects the facial muscles. Intraoperatively, it can be identified as a shiny fibrous layer located between the dermis and deep fascial muscles. Superiorly the SMAS is densely adherent to the zygomatic arch and the temporalis fascia and inferiorly interdigitates with the dermis in the cheek, platysma over the mandible, and the sternomastoid muscle fascia in the neck. The motor branches of the facial nerve lie deep to the SMAS. Because of its bony and soft tissue attachments, the SMAS acts as an important distributor of facial muscular contractions to the skin.

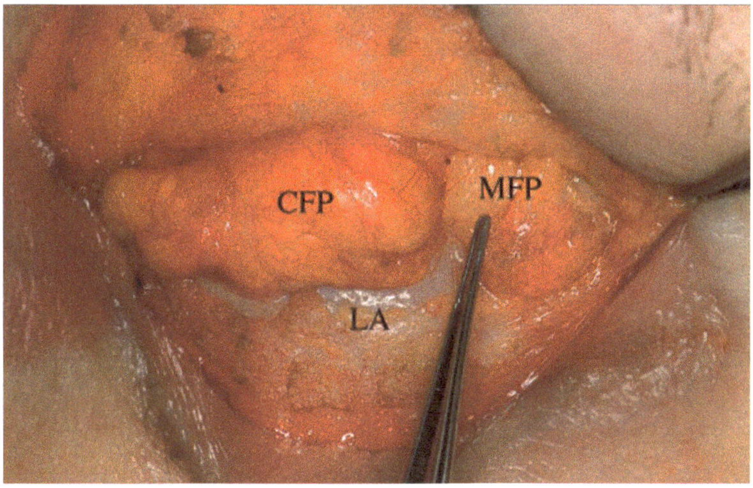


**Fig. 1.4** Intraoperative photo of the upper lid fat pads demonstrates a central and medial fat pad (CFP, MFP). There is no lateral fat pad in the upper lid, and lateral fullness would indicate lacrimal gland prolapse

The soft tissues of the face can be considered as layers similar to the scalp—skin, subcutaneous connective tissue, musculoaponeurotic (SMAS), loose areolar tissue and space, and periosteum. The musculoaponeurotic layer, or SMAS, is attached to the dermis of the skin via fine reticular fibers from the subcutaneous tissues and invests the intrinsic muscles of the face. The areolar tissue contains the facial ligaments that are the pillars of attachment between the soft tissue and the bony skeleton. The main ligaments in the cheek region are the orbicularis retaining (orbitomalar), zygomatic, and masseteric ligaments. Free spaces can be found between the ligaments where there is no attachment of the soft tissue to underlying bone, thus creating glide planes that become prominent with aging. The midcheek has compact ligament attachments bonding the large soft tissue area to the underlying bony surface.

It is also important to understand that the lamellar arrangement of facial muscles is crucial to providing firm facial tissue support, as well as influencing the contour and expressions of the face. The most superficial layer consists of the frontalis, orbicularis oculi, zygomaticus minor, and the depressor anguli oris; the second layer comprises the depressor supercilii, zygomaticus major, levator labii superioris, alaeque nasi, depressor labii inferioris, and platysma; and the third layer consists of the levator labii superioris and orbicularis oris. The deepest layer includes the corrugator supercilii, mentalis, levator anguli oris, and buccinator muscles.

In recent years, there has also been more interest in the aesthetic implications of various facial and periocular fat pads. It is understood that the fat structures of the face are crucial in recreating the youthful appearance of the face and need to be restored carefully in specific regions. The topography of these fat structures forms the basis of facial contouring with harvested fat or soft tissue fillers.

The two upper and three lower eyelid fat pads are located posterior to the septum and ideally should not be debulked posteriorly past the orbital rim border in order to avoid the hollow socket appearance (Fig. 1.4). A fat pad posterior to the eyebrow, known as the retroorbicularis oculi fat (ROOF), provides structural support for the eyebrow. When correcting brow ptosis in women, the ROOF should be secured to the periosteum approximately one to two centimeters above the supraorbital rim.

The midface or malar fat lies typically over and medial to the malar eminence of the upper cheek. The location of these structures along with the shape of the face should be considered when planning the injection of fillers aimed at lifting

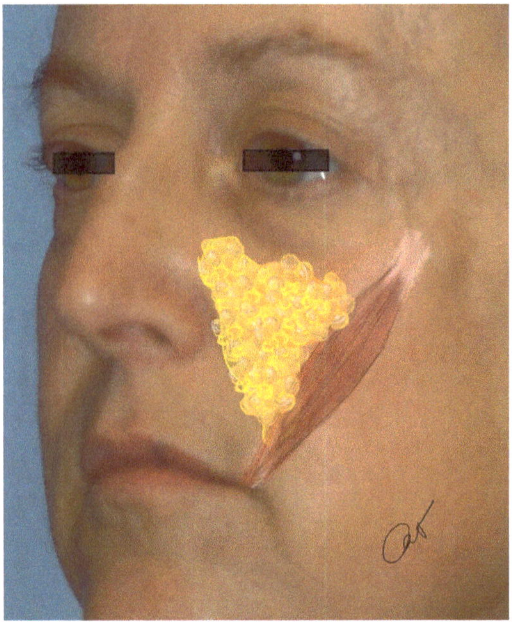

**Fig. 1.5** Deep medial cheek fat along the medial border of the zygomaticus major muscle. This is an important anatomical space while injecting dermal fillers and should be augmented properly in order to recreate a youthful anterior projection to the midface and tear trough

the malar and medial cheek regions (Fig. 1.5). The suborbicularis oculi fat (SOOF) [15] is located beneath the orbicularis oculi plane of the lower lid and is separated from the periorbital fat by the thin orbital and malar septum. Malar fat pads, located below the orbital margin level, can descend with ptosis of the SOOF. The sub-SMAS fat in the malar region is continuous with the sub-muscular fat in the eyebrow region. The buccal fat lies deep in the face and comprises buccal, temporal, and pterygoid extensions [16].

## Forehead and Glabella

The upper face can be considered as a cosmetic unit that comprises the forehead, glabella, and eyebrows. The forehead runs superiorly from the anterior hairline to the zygoma laterally and the brows inferiorly [17]. The intersection of the forehead frontal bone with the nasal bones caudally on each side of the midline is referred to as the nation. The forehead can also be divided into

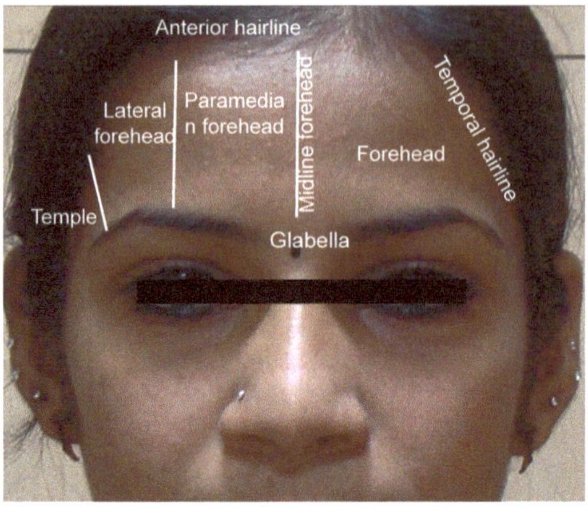


**Fig. 1.6** Anatomical divisions of the forehead

midline forehead, paramedian forehead, lateral forehead, temporal, and brow regions (Fig. 1.6). There is a gentle smooth rounded convex contour from the midline to the midbrow area that becomes flatter laterally towards the more concave temporal region. The forehead is a multilayered structure that comprises, from anterior to posterior, the skin, subcutaneous connective tissue, muscle, galea aponeurotica, loose areolar tissue and glide space, and periosteum (Fig. 1.7).

Facial skin is thickest on the forehead and is relatively inelastic and immobile centrally, although increases in mobility laterally. The galea aponeurotica is a broad musculoaponeurotic layer that is firmly attached to the occipital protuberance posteriorly and fuses with the superficial temporalis fascia laterally which continues with the SMAS in the cheek and neck. The loose areolar tissue posterior to the forehead muscles and galea permit movement of the scalp over the periosteum. The galea aponeurotica divides into a superficial and deep layer to envelope the paired frontalis muscles. The superficial layer covers the anterior frontalis muscle surface, and the deep layer traverses posteriorly to merge along the supraorbital rim into the arcus marginalis and postorbicular fascial plane of the eyelids [18].

The forehead musculature comprises mainly the frontalis muscle. The glabellar muscle complex includes the corrugator supercilii (CSM), depressor supercilii (DSM), and procerus

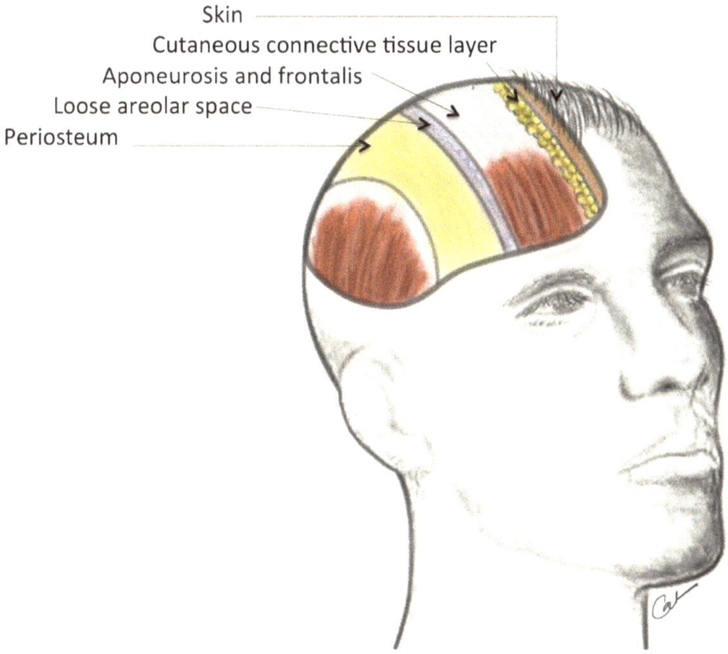


**Fig. 1.7** Tissue layers of the scalp and face consist of, from anterior to posterior, the skin, cutaneous connective tissue, aponeurosis (including frontalis and SMAS of the face), loose areolar space and glide planes, and periosteum

muscles (Fig. 1.8). The superficial group of muscles involved in the formation of glabellar rhytids includes the frontalis, procerus, and orbicularis oculi muscles; the intermediate group includes the depressor supercilii muscles; and the deep group is composed of the corrugator supercilii muscles. Vertical lines of the glabella are caused primarily by the transverse head of the corrugator supercilii muscle. Horizontal rhytids are a result of hyperactive procerus, oblique head of the corrugator, and depressor supercilii muscles; and oblique lines are caused by the transverse head of the corrugator supercilii and the medial orbicularis oculi fibers [19, 20].

## Frontalis Muscle

The frontalis muscle is the main muscle mass of the forehead and lies beneath the subcutaneous tissue plane. It is the primary elevator of the forehead and eyebrows and is an accessory elevator of the eyelids. Its antagonist muscles are the eyebrow depressor group (Fig. 1.9).

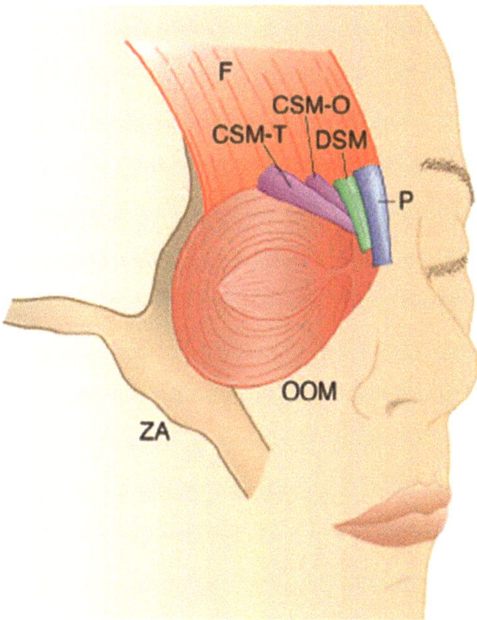


**Fig. 1.8** Schematic diagram of the anatomical locations and relations of the glabellar and brow musculature (*CSM-O* corrugator supercilii muscle oblique head, *CSM-T* corrugator supercilii muscle transverse head, *DSM* depressor supercilii muscle, *F* frontalis, *OOM* orbital orbicularis oculi, *P* procerus, *ZA* zygomatic arch)

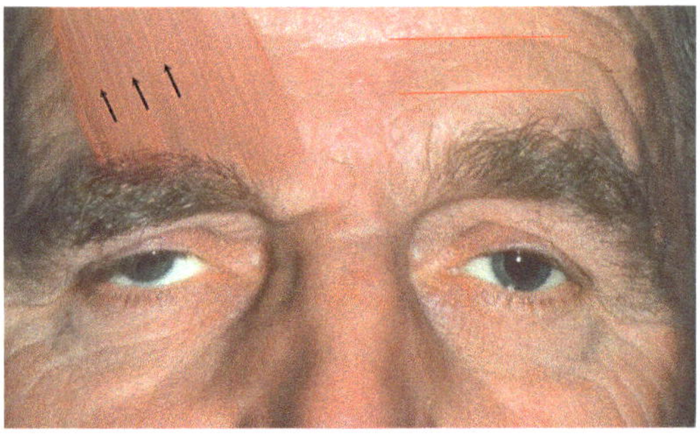

**Fig. 1.9** Anatomical overlay of frontalis muscle action. The frontalis muscle is the primary elevator of the forehead and brows (*arrows*). Muscle contraction leads to formation of deep transverse forehead lines (*lines*)

The frontalis is an approximately 7 cm quadrilateral muscle originating from the galea aponeurotica along the coronal suture line. It expands over the frontal bone without bony attachment and inserts into the dermis of the brow skin inferiorly. Laterally the muscle fibers extend slightly higher than the medial fibers and fuse at or just lateral to the temporal fusion line. The muscle interdigitates inferiorly with the eyebrow depressor muscles, which include the CSM, DSM, orbicularis oculi, and procerus muscles. Multiple transverse-oriented septa extending from the dermis to the frontalis muscle have been demonstrated, suggesting that continuous contraction of the frontalis muscle fibers and the transverse septa leads to the formation of deep transverse forehead lines or rhytides with increased aging [21].

Classically the frontalis muscle has been described as two distinct and separate oblique bellies in the forehead, leaving the central forehead region devoid of muscle. However, reports of a single broad belly have also been documented [22]. This anatomical variation often leads to the presence of variable functional patterns of frontalis contraction. For instance, patients presenting with a deep transverse contiguous line likely have a single broad frontalis muscle without separation or two large wider muscles, and therefore chemodenervation in these patients may be tailored to include focal injections in the central forehead as well. Others may present with distinct arches above each brow laterally while the central forehead remains flat. Dissection in these patients may reveal two separate frontalis muscle bellies.

## Procerus

The procerus muscle is a main depressor of the medial eyebrow and originates as a thin triangular muscle from the periosteum of the nasal bone to insert vertically in the dermis of the glabella or midforehead between the medial frontalis muscle bellies. It lies in the same plane as the frontalis muscle and is the most superficial muscle of the eyebrow depressors. Contraction of the procerus pulls the medial eyebrow inferiorly and slightly medially, which produces the common transverse wrinkles over the nasal bridge. Motor innervation is supplied by the frontal branch, and sometimes the buccal branch, of the facial nerve.

## Depressor Supercilii Muscles

The paired depressor supercilii muscles originate approximately 1 cm above the medial canthus from the periosteum of the frontal bone and insert tangentially into the dermis of each medial eyebrow. The DSM is the intermediate muscle group of the eyebrow depressors and lies deep to the procerus muscle and anterior to the CSM. Other authors have suggested these muscle fibers are part of the corrugator or orbicularis oculi muscles, rather than a distinct muscle. A simple way to visualize the depressor supercilii is that it is the muscle that runs lateral to the procerus. It is typically innervated by the temporal branch of the facial nerve and acts as an accessory depressor of the medial eyebrow.

## Corrugator Supercilii Muscles

The CSM are also secondary eyebrow depressors and are the deepest layer of muscles, located posterior to the procerus and DSM. They originate from the nasal process of the frontal bone and travel obliquely superiorly and laterally over the supraorbital rim between the bellies of the frontalis

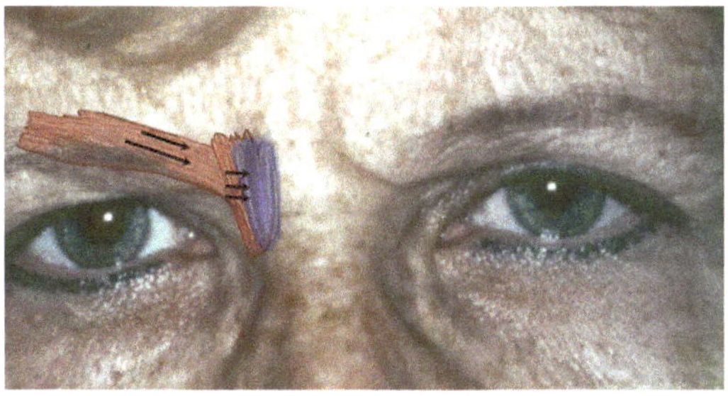

**Fig. 1.10** The depressor supercilii muscle and the oblique and transverse heads of the corrugator supercilii muscle (*red*) act as depressors of the eyebrow. Contraction of these depressor muscles, including the procerus muscle, results in oblique, vertical, and horizontal rhytids of the glabella

and the medial orbicularis muscle to insert into the dermis of the medial and midbrow. It is deep centrally and becomes superficial laterally. It typically ends approximately 1.7–3.0 cm lateral to the glabellar midline, although some studies have found extension of the CSM as far as the lateral aspect of the eyebrow. Patients should be asked to frown in order to visualize the most lateral extension of these muscles, since cosmetic botulinum toxin injections would therefore be customized to neutralize this lateral muscle. The CSM insertions lie approximately 30° above horizontal, which results in the CSM functioning as both an eyebrow apposer (to draw the medial brows together) and a depressor. The corrugator muscle is typically supplied by the temporal branch of the facial nerve.

The corrugator has two distinct muscle heads, called the transverse and oblique heads. The oblique head originates from the superior part of the medial orbital rim along with the DSM and inserts as a short square-like muscle into the medial brow dermis. The transverse head originates from the medial part of the superior orbital rim and travels farther and more horizontally to insert into the medial third to half of the eyebrow. As a result of the anatomy, contraction of the vertical oblique muscle head clinically manifests as the horizontal or oblique glabellar frown lines, whereas contraction of the transverse heads pulls the brows more medially and results in vertical glabellar creases (Fig. 1.10). As mentioned previously, having the patient frown with the eyebrows can illustrate where the lateral insertions of the transverse CSM are located, which are seen as dimpling or pulling of the skin just above the mid-eyebrow hairs. The injections sites for chemodenervation would thus include the lateral muscle edges in order to achieve maximal results. Care must be taken to avoid injecting too far above the eyebrow hairs, however, as this could weaken the inferior frontalis muscle instead, resulting in iatrogenic brow ptosis.

## Orbicularis Oculi

The orbicularis oculi is one of the major muscles of facial expression, acting as the eyelid protractor and an accessory depressor of the forehead. It has a characteristic circular configuration around the upper and lower eyelids, with multiple insertions into the eyelid skin that often makes surgical separation between these two tissue planes difficult. The orbicularis oculi has been further divided topographically into the pretarsal portion which lies anterior to the tarsal plates, the preseptal muscle overlying the orbital septum, and the orbital portion overlying the superior and inferior orbital rims.

The thick orbital fibers arise from the medial canthal tendon, arch horizontally and concentrically along the orbital rims to meet laterally at the zygoma. The medial and superior parts of the orbital fibers of the orbicularis muscle interdigitate superiorly with the frontalis muscle fibers, DSM, and lateral procerus. Contraction of the orbital orbicularis muscle thus pulls the skin of the forehead, brow, and cheeks towards the eye and leads to the formation of oblique glabellar lines. Laterally, the vertically oriented orbicularis fibers depress the lateral brow and create the "crow's feet" lines with aging. Cosmetic chemodenervation of the lateral orbital orbicularis fibers may also achieve subtle lateral brow elevation by weakening the brow depressor action of the muscle.

The thinner preseptal orbicularis fibers also originate at the medial canthal tendon and meet laterally to contribute to the lateral palpebral raphe. The pretarsal fibers are firmly adherent to the tarsus and travel in an elliptical path adjacent to the eyelid margins. Medially, the pretarsal

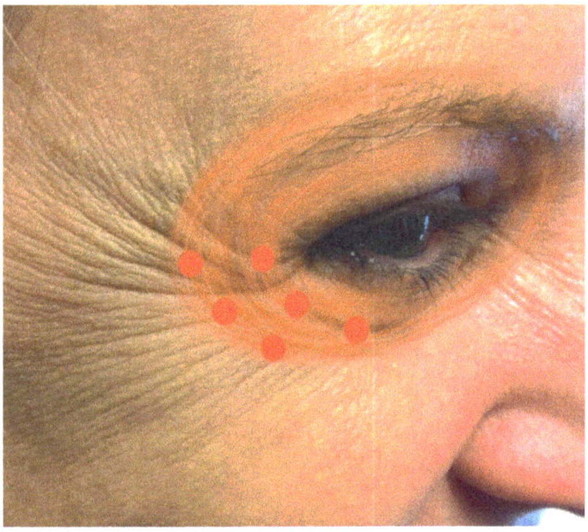

**Fig. 1.11** Contraction of the vertical fibers of the lateral orbicularis oculi muscle leads to characteristic horizontal creases that expand outwards from the lateral canthus. These orbicularis muscle fibers can be treated with botulinum toxin injections for diminishing periocular lines

orbicularis splits into superficial and deep heads, with the deep head arising from the posterior lacrimal crest. Laterally, the pretarsal orbicularis also forms superficial and deep heads which contribute to the lateral canthal tendon [16]. The preseptal orbicularis supports the orbital septum, especially during smiling, and may also play a role in lymphatic drainage. Traditionally it was thought that weakening of the preseptal orbicularis and orbital septum may contribute to age-related lower eyelid fullness and fat prolapse. The various orbicularis oculi muscle portions are innervated by the temporal or zygomatic branches of the facial nerve, with some muscle portions receiving dual innervation. Contraction of the vertical lateral orbicularis oculi muscle, including the orbital portion of the orbicularis muscle, results in horizontal and oblique lateral skin rhytids along the lateral raphe and upper cheek. These dynamic creases are amenable to treatment with botulinum toxin, targeting these vertical orbicularis oculi muscle fibers lateral to the orbital rim (Fig. 1.11).

## Eyebrows

The eyebrows play a crucial role in facial expression, with their position dependent upon an interplay of elevators and depressors [23, 24].

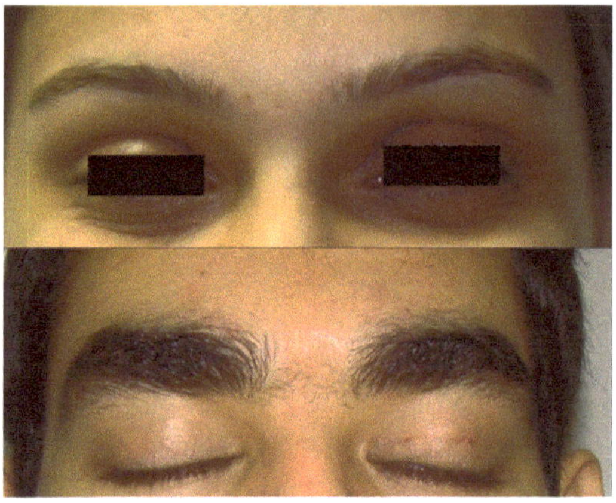

**Fig. 1.12** Ideal topography of a female and male brow

The frontalis muscle, which interdigitates with the orbicularis muscle in the region of the eyebrows, is the sole elevator of the brow, whereas the eyebrow depressors include the glabellar complex which was discussed previously.

The head of the brow lies at the medial supraorbital ridge; the body of the brow follows the supraorbital margin; and the tail overlies the lateral angular process of frontal bone and extends up to the zygomaticofrontal suture. It is broadest nasally and narrows laterally. Topographically, an ideal female brow arches approximately 1 cm above the supraorbital rim with the maximum height at the lateral canthus or two-thirds laterally, whereas a male brow is typically more flat and lies lower at the level of the supraorbital rim [25] (Fig. 1.12). Variations as well as ethnic differences in regard to the height and contour of the eyebrow should always be considered in the preoperative evaluation.

The soft tissue layers at the eyebrow consist, from anterior to posterior, of hair-bearing skin, muscle, fat, aponeurosis (galea), and periosteum. The galea aponeurotica envelops the frontalis muscle superiorly in the forehead, and as it traverses towards the brow, envelops the brow fat pad and also serves as a glide plane posterior to the fat pad to allow for eyebrow movement. The skin of the brow consists of numerous sweat and sebaceous glands, and the cilia are more angulated at the medial brow compared to the lateral brow hairs. The upper rows of cilia grow down and laterally, while the lower cilia grow up and laterally.

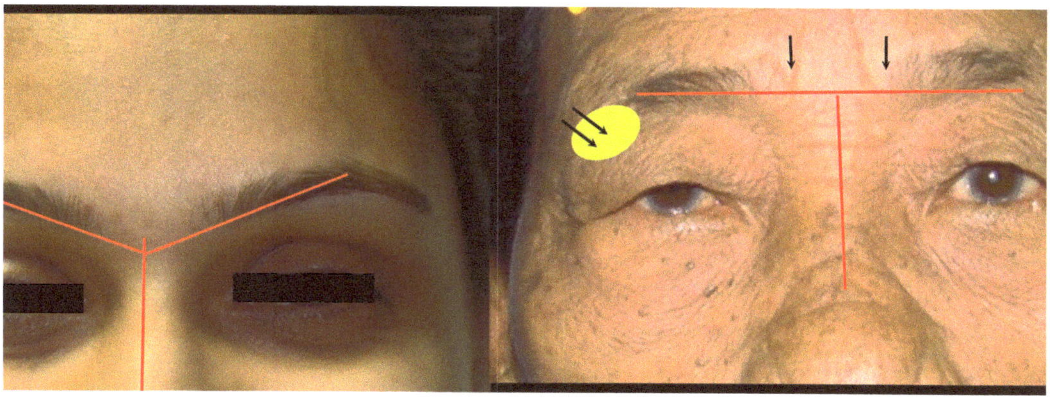

**Fig. 1.13** With aging the eyebrow falls below the supraorbital rim secondary to the ROOF descent (*yellow with arrows*) and forehead ptosis (*black arrows*). Note the change in the nasal eyebrow angle from the youthful Y-configuration to an aged T-configuration

The eyebrow fat pad, or retroorbicularis oculi fat (ROOF) pad, contributes to lateral eyebrow volume and youthful periorbital fullness. The ROOF is continuous with the posterior orbicularis fascia in the eyelid [26] and extends into the eyelid septum through its posterior fascial extension. With aging, a descended ROOF into the eyelid space should not be mistaken for prolapsed orbital fat, but instead should be elevated rather than excised and secured over the orbital rim. The fat pad may also atrophy, and therefore meticulous volume augmentation over the periosteum of the lateral and superior orbital rim may restore the youthful rounded appearance below the brows, as well as elevate the lateral brow position.

Habitual eyebrow elevation may often occur as a natural compensatory response to blepharoptosis and dermatochalasis. With aging, however, the eyebrow falls below the supraorbital rim, which can contribute to additional visual field obstruction, and the nasal eyebrow angle changes from the youthful Y-configuration to an aged T-configuration (Fig. 1.13). Lateral brow ptosis is often the initial manifestation of age-related changes and is anatomically due to lack of the frontalis muscle extending and inserting into the lateral portion of the brows. Therefore, as involutional changes occur with age, including atrophy of the brow fat pad and gravitational pull, brow ptosis occurs and frontalis contraction compensates to lift the eyebrow and eyelids. As there is typically no or minimal frontalis muscle laterally, this manifests clinically as lateral eyebrow ptosis. Facial rejuvenation procedures should therefore elevate the lateral brow more than the medial brow to restore the youthful appearance. Botulinum toxin injections to the lateral vertically oriented orbital orbicularis oculi muscle fibers adjacent to the lateral canthal angle may also help weaken the unopposed downward pull of the lateral brow to help reestablish lateral brow elevation.

## Midface

The upper cheek fullness and rounded contour of the midface denotes youthfulness; therefore, when the midface descends and loses its natural volume over time, the face appears aged and tired. Schematically, the midface can be defined as the area encompassed by an imaginary line drawn above the zygomatic arch from just below the superior helix insertion to the lateral canthus and a lower line that extends from the inferior tragal cartilage to below the oral commissure [27].

The midcheek region of the midface is a triangular area between the lower eyelid and the nasolabial fold inferiorly. Medially, the midcheek blends with the lateral nasal border. The outer border of the midcheek is continuous with the lateral cheek around the prominence over the zygoma.

The surface of the bony midface is formed by the zygoma and the anterior surface of the maxilla, which provide points of attachment for the

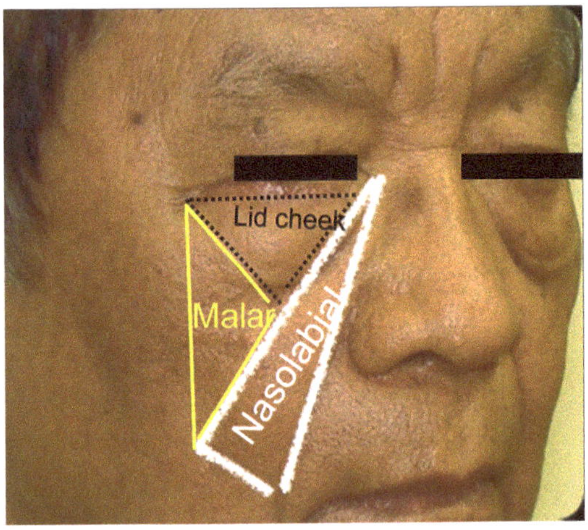


**Fig. 1.14** Schematic components of the midface

muscles of the lower lid, lip, and other facial ligaments to support the midface. The midface can be considered as being comprised of three main sections: the lid-cheek segment, the malar segment, and the nasolabial segment (Fig. 1.14). These segments are separated by the palpebromalar groove superolaterally, nasojugal groove medially, and the midcheek furrow inferiorly. The lid-cheek segment has no defined boundaries or bony attachments, but in youth typically lies above the level of the inferior orbital rim. The contour of this region of the midface has often been described as a smooth convexity seen on lateral oblique views. With involutional changes, the single rounded contour separates into two continuous convex shapes ("double-convexity deformity") as the lower lid fat prolapses and the midfacial tissues descend below the orbital rim, resulting in a clinical appearance of eyelid and cheek separation (Fig. 1.15). The valley between the two convexities is referred to as the tear trough or nasojugal deformity and is often augmented with soft tissue fillers, fat repositioning, or fat transfer to restore the single convexity of youth. It is also important to understand that the thickness of the midfacial skin changes and becomes thinner as it approaches the rim and eyelid; therefore, placement of volume augmentation should be minimized or avoided posterior to the thin eyelid skin as there is significantly increased risk of lumpiness and Tyndall effect.

In addition to the change in contour of the lid-cheek segment, aging signs also manifest in the skin itself, such as increased static lines and rhytids, solar pigmentation, increased telangiectasias or spider veins, increased laxity, and dullness to the skin. These changes can be corrected with chemical peels, laser resurfacing, or intense pulsed light treatments as mentioned previously.

The malar segment is a triangular-shaped area bordered by the lid-cheek segment superomedially, nasolabial fold inferomedially, and the temple and lateral face laterally. The prezygomatic space anteriorly to the maxillary process of the zygoma is bordered by ligamentous attachments—the orbicularis retaining ligament (orbitomalar ligament) superiorly and the zygomatic ligaments inferiorly, which play an important role in facial aging. The suborbicularis oculi fat (SOOF) layer posterior to the lower eyelid orbicularis oculi muscle is analogous to the eyebrow ROOF fat layer and is often repositioned superiorly over the malar eminence to rejuvenate the midface [28, 29].

The nasolabial segment extends from the side of the nose medially to the malar segment laterally [30]. It is defined laterally by the nasojugal fold. The inferior aspect of the nasolabial segment overlies the vestibule of the oral cavity. The lateral portion is anchored by the zygomatic and the masseteric ligaments. The subcutaneous tissue of this segment is thicker and more mobile when compared to the other segments of the midface. The space beneath the outer part of the nasolabial segment contains the buccal fat pads [31]. With aging, this portion of the midface descends below the oral commissure which creates fullness in the lower face and deepening of the nasolabial fold [32]. Bony absorption of the maxilla and zygoma with age manifesting as loss of volume projection of the midface and attenuation of the ligamentous supports contribute to flattening of the normally rounded midcheek and the development of mid- and lower facial furrows. Therefore, ideal facial rejuvenation procedures combine elevation of the descended fat pads with support of the attenuated facial ligaments, in addition of augmentation of lost volume.

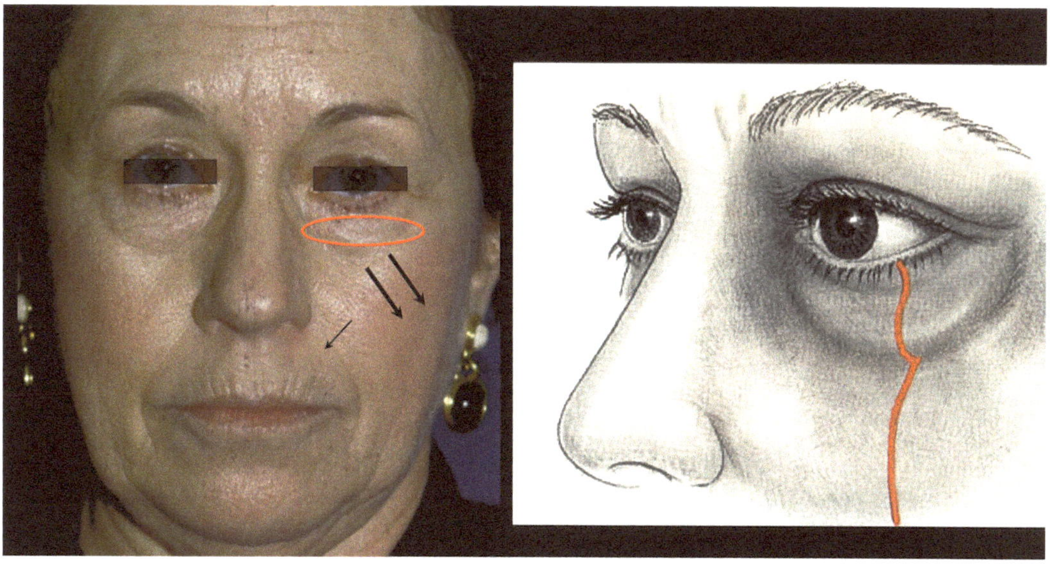

**Fig. 1.15** Facial aging demonstrated by a prominent tear trough deformity (*red circle*) and deep nasolabial folds secondary to midfacial ptosis and descent. On lateral profile, the classic double-convexity contour is a result of eyelid and cheek separation and greater visibility of the bony inferior orbital rim

## Conclusion

The anatomy of the face and eyelid is complex and is continuing to be better understood in relation to the aging process. Only with a thorough knowledge of detailed anatomy and its practical aspects can optimal results of a procedure be achieved.

## References


1. Pendergast PM. Facial proportions. In: Erian A, Shiffman MA, editors. Advanced surgical facial rejuvenation; Springer 2012. p. 15–22.
2. Tolleth H. Concepts for the plastic surgeon from art and sculpture. Clin Plast Surg. 1987;14(4):585–98.
3. Vegter F, Hage J. Clinical anthropometry and canons of the face in historical perspective. Plast Reconstr Surg. 2000;106(5):1090–6.
4. Ricketts RM. The golden divider. J Clin Orthod. 1981;15(11):752–9.
5. Ricketts RM. Divine proportion in facial aesthetics. Clin Plast Surg. 1982;9(4):401–22.
6. Lee JH, Kim TG, Park GW, Kim YH. Cumulative frequency distribution in East Asian facial widths using the facial golden mask. J Craniofac Surg. 2009;20(5):1378–82.
7. Marquardt SR, Stephen R. Marquardt on the Golden Decagon and human facial beauty. Interview by Dr. Gottlieb. J Clin Orthodont. 2002;36:339–47.
8. Ruess W, Owsley JQ. The anatomy of the skin and fascial layers of the face in aesthetic surgery. Clin Plast Surg. 1987;14:677–82.
9. Glogau R. Physiologic and structural changes associated with aging skin. Dermatol Clin. 1997;15:555–9.
10. Carruthers J, Cohen SR, Joseph JH, Narins RS, Rubin M. The science and art of dermal fillers for soft-tissue augmentation. J Drugs Dermatol. 2009;8(4):335–50.
11. Arletti JP, Trotter MJ. Anatomic location of hyaluronic acid filler material injected into nasolabial fold: a histologic study. Dermatol Surg. 2008;34:s56–63.
12. Hatton MP. Rubin PA review of facial anatomy as it relates to the use of botulinum toxin. Int Ophthalmol Clin. 2005;45:37–9.
13. Bhertha TM. Facial anatomy and the application of fillers and botulinum toxin - Part I. Surg Cosmet Dermatol. 2010;2(3):195–204.
14. Mitz V, Peyronie M. The superficial musculoaponeurotic system (SMAS) in the parotid and cheek area. Plast Reconstr Surg. 1976;58:80–8.
15. Hoenig JA, Shorr N, Shorr J. The suborbicularis oculi fat in aesthetic and reconstructive surgery. Int Ophthalmol Clin. 1997;37:179–91.
16. Sires BS, Lemke BN, Dortzbach RK, Gonnering RS. Characterization of human orbital fat and connective tissue. Ophthal Plast Reconstr Surg. 1998;14:403–14.
17. Vuyk HD. Forehead, temple and scalp reconstruction. http://www.vuyk.nl/publicaties/nr/034.pdf.
18. Lemke BN, Stasior OG. The anatomy of eyebrow ptosis. Arch Ophthalmol. 1982;100:981–6.

19. Burkat CN, Lucarelli MJ, Lemke BN. Comprehensive glabellar anatomy for the cosmetic surgeon. Am J Cosmetic Surg. 2005;22:7–24.
20. Ellis DA, Bakala CD. Anatomy of the motor innervation of the corrugator supercilii muscle: clinical significance and development of a new surgical technique for frowning. J Otolaryngol. 1998;27:222–7.
21. Tan TS, Oh S-R, Priel A, Korn BS, Kikkawa DO. Surgical anatomy of the forehead, eyelids, and midface for the aesthetic surgeon. In: Massry GG, Murphy MR, Azizzadeh B, editors. Master techniques in blepharoplasty and periorbital rejuvenation. NY, USA: Springer; 2011. doi:10.1007/978-1-4614-0067-7_2.
22. Finn JC. Practical botulinum toxin anatomy - Finn facial plastics, SE Cox- http://www.finnface.com
23. Lemke BN, Stasior OG. Eyebrow incision making. Ophthal Plast Reconstr Surg. 1983;2:19–23.
24. Knize D. An anatomically based study of the mechanism of eyebrow ptosis. Plast Reconstr Surg. 1996;97:1321–33.
25. Freund RM, Nolan III WB. Correlation between brow lift outcomes and aesthetic ideals for eyebrow height and shape in females. Plast Reconstr Surg. 1996;97:1343–8.
26. Putterman AM, Urist MJ. Surgical anatomy of the orbital septum. Ann Ophthalmol. 1974;6:290–4.
27. Rohrich RJ, Pessa JE, Ristow B. The youthful cheek and the deep medial fat compartment. Plast Reconstr Surg. 2008;121:2107–12.
28. Kikkawa DO, Lemke BN, Dortzbach RK. Relations of the superficial musculoaponeurotic system to the orbit and characterization of the orbitomalar ligament. Ophthal Plast Reconstr Surg. 1996;12:77–88.
29. Furnas DW. The retaining ligaments of the cheek. Plast Reconstr Surg. 1989;83:11–6.
30. Barton FE. The SMAS and the nasolabial fold. Plast Reconstr Surg. 1992;89:1054–9.
31. Stuzin JM, Wagstrom L, Kawamoto HK, Baker TJ, Wolfe SA. The anatomy and clinical applications of the buccal fat pad. Plast Reconstr Surg. 1990;85:29–37.
32. Lucarelli MJ, Khwarg SI, Lemke BN, Kozel JS, Dortzbach RK. The anatomy of midfacial ptosis. Ophthal Plast Reconstr Surg. 2000;16:7–22.

# Neuromodulators: Contemporary Indications and Techniques in the Upper and Midface

2

Corey S. Maas

## Brief History of Botulinum Neurotoxin and Aesthetic Indications

Early use of Botulinum toxin (Fig. 2.1) can be credited to ophthalmologist Dr. Allen Scott who communicated to the senior author and other in the late 1980s and early 1990s his observations of wrinkle effacement when treating blepharospasm [1]. These observations led to early reports of Botulinum toxins employed to target specifically hyperfunctional frown lines [2]. The great success of this molecule in aesthetic applications can thus be credited to the innovative thinking and initiative of clinicians with interest in advancing clinical care in contrast to the more common pharmaceutical-based, profit-motivated development of drugs and devices.

Thus, Allergan, Inc. (Irvine, CA) must credit this physician-lead curiosity and clinical initiative with taking a little known orphan drug, Botox™ to what is now known as Botox Cosmetic™ (roughly $25 million to over one billion in annual sales). More importantly, the use of this molecule in aesthetic and reconstructive surgery has changed the contemporary approach to patients in complimentary fields.

The Botulinum toxins are naturally occurring complex proteins (heavy and light chain dimers) that in nature are surrounded by "inactive" complexing proteins. It should be noted that research presented at Toxins 2012 (Miami, FL, 2012) shows activity in membrane penetration and/or permeability related to these complexing proteins and their function is, at best, poorly understood. Such properties may explain subtle differences in clinical characteristics of the various BoNTA products. The "active" heavy and light chains are responsible for neuronal terminal end uptake and cleavage of proteins responsible for acetylcholine vesicle release into the neurosynaptic cleft, respectively [3].

Terminology in medicine is important and heretofore the protein basic science community has referred to the Botulinum toxins simply as "toxins" and has developed an industry standard abbreviation, by consensus, of BoNTA and BoNTB for the commercially available A and B serotypes of Botulinum toxins, respectively. While terms like "toxin" work for basic science community, referring to these medications (or any medications for that matter) in discussions with patients would be unnecessarily alarming and, in principle, inaccurate.

In practice all medications are "toxins" in large or incorrect dosages. This has led many clinicians to adopt (appropriately in the author's opinion) alternative terminologies when describing this

Electronic supplementary material The online version of this chapter (doi:10.1007/978-1-4614-8388-5_2) contains supplementary material, which is available to authorized users.

C.S. Maas, M.D., F.A.C.S. (✉)
The Maas Clinic, University of California,
San Francisco, San Francisco, CA, USA
e-mail: drmaas@maasclinic.com

S.A. Myint (ed.), *Nonsurgical Peri-orbital Rejuvenation*, DOI 10.1007/978-1-4614-8388-5_2,

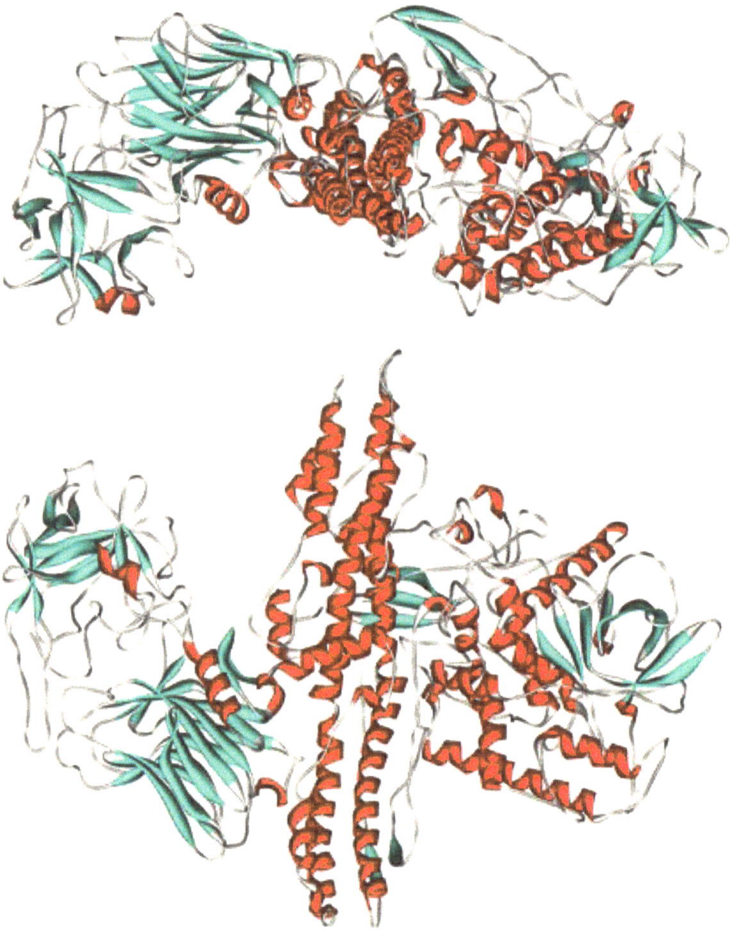

**Fig. 2.1** Botulinum toxin protein

class of medications. Ideally, industry or a representative group of clinician thought leaders would meet and agree upon an appropriate standard clinical nomenclature. For now it appears the term "neuromodulator" seems to have gained acceptance. As defined by Mosby's Medical Dictionary a *neuromodulator is "a substance that alters nerve impulse transmission"* [4]. While certain industry and clinician spokespersons have claimed to have "invented" the term neuromodulator, it is hardly a new term and such claims have generated controversy around the adoption of this term. For purposes of this chapter we will refer to the clinically available forms of Botulinum neurotoxin BoNT as neuromodulators (NMs).

## Introduction of New NMs and Relevant Dosages

While Botox Cosmetic™ has become a mainstay workhorse and household name other relevant competitors have been introduced with varying success.

Myobloc™ (US WorldMeds, S. San Francisco, CA) the only B serotype neuromodulator is supplied in a sterile slightly acidic and stable solution ready for injection. Its efficacy and use in neurology was not found in clinical studies to be effective for aesthetic applications due to its shorter clinical effect and pain on injection [5, 6].

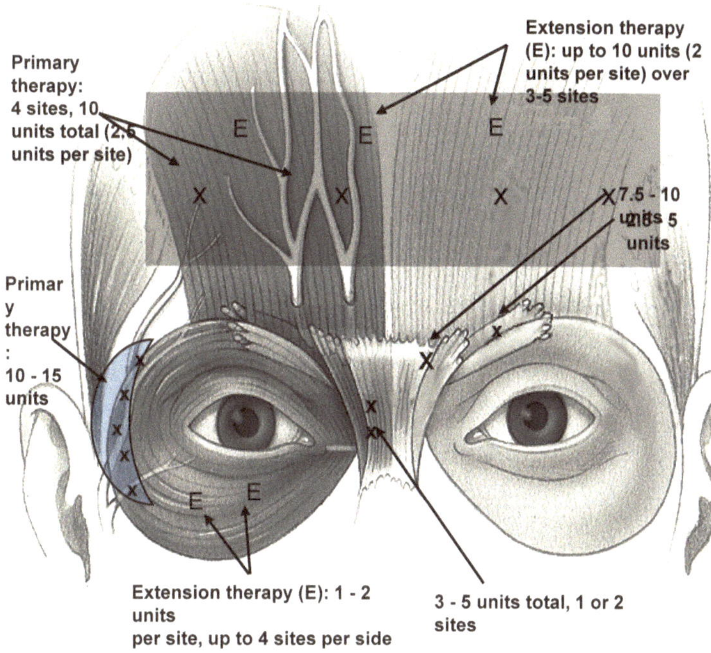


**Fig. 2.2** BoTox cosmetic injection sites and dosages

Effectively the US market has currently three available forms of BoNTA and one under FDA consideration.

Each of these products is provided in a dry form with instructions for reconstitution in sterile saline. Many clinicians prefer the use of preserved saline with reports of decreased pain on injection. The author uses normal saline. With slightly greater area of effect with Dysport™ (Medicis Corp Scottsdale, AZ), we use smaller volumes of diluent (1.5 ml) than with Botox (2.0 ml). Reported ranges in clinical use for diluent volume are generally accepted to be between 1.0 and 4.0 ml. The lower end volumes require very small and incremental injections and may be difficult to effectively cover larger muscle groups and the higher end volumes result in more local swelling and potentially diffusion-related side effects. This has not been proven to our knowledge in controlled trials, however, and it is advised that the clinician uses the mid range of diluent volumes.

Since its cosmetic indication market clearance in 2002 (and before) Botox Cosmetic™ remains the industry standard and its applications have expanded well beyond the early upper face indications [7, 8]. It is supplied as a lyophilized powder and the company has gone to great lengths to reduce the worldwide problem with forgery and false product distribution (often over the Internet) with the use of holograms and Botox Cosmetic™ product-specific identifiers.

Consistency in potency and clinical results as well as its established trade name are strong benefits of Botox Cosmetic™. The points of injection and dosages employed by the author are shown in Fig. 2.2.

Dysport™ was FDA-cleared in 2009 with a slow adoption curve largely due to overdosage in the frontalis muscle and resultant brow ptosis. This product has proven to be an excellent competitor for Botox Cosmetic™ and its wider area of effect can be harnessed to provide more effective rhytid effacement in the flatter orbicularis and frontalis muscle groups. A split face double blind study comparing Botox Cosmetic™ and Dysport for lateral orbital rhytids at 10 and 30 units, respectively, showed a 2:1 (61 of 90 patients) preferred the Dysport™ treatment side with a 17 % greater improvement over Botox Cosmetic™ at 1 and 3 months post-treatment [9]. The author's treatment points and dosages are shown in Fig. 2.3.

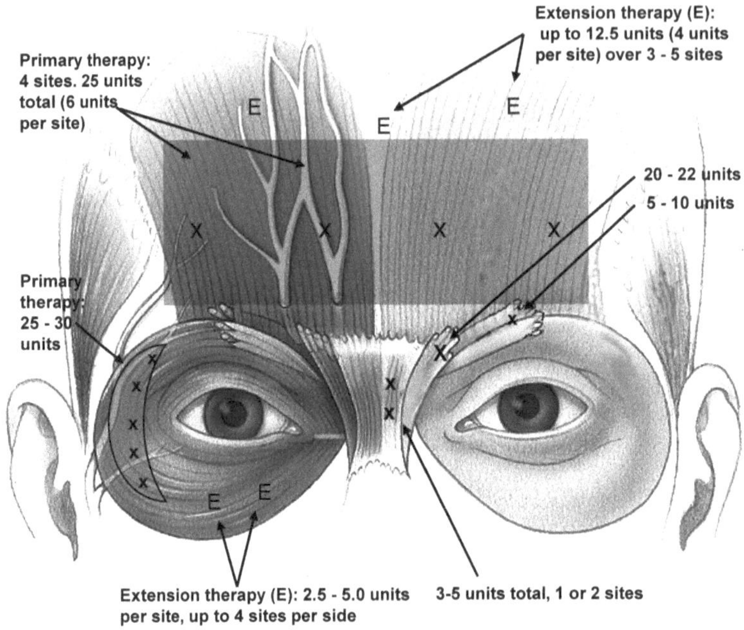


**Fig. 2.3** DYSPORT injection sites and dosage

While individual products cannot be directly compared on a unit for unit basis most experienced clinicians are using Botox Unit (BU) to Dysport Unit (DU) ratio of 2.5 or 3:1. Stated another way, 20 BU is roughly the same in performance characteristics as 50–60 BU. We noted early after release of Dysport that 25 unit dosing showed rapid onset but early clinical effectiveness decay at or before 12 weeks in the glabella. In contrast, consistently greater than 12 weeks duration was seen at the 60 unit dosage for glabellar furrows. Apparently there was a reason Ipsen, Inc. (London, UK) produces Dysport in 300 unit vials (vs. 100 unit vials for Botox or 3:1).

Xeomin™ (Merz Aesthetics, Greensboro, NC) has proprietary manufacturing that *removes* the aforementioned "inactive" proteins which was thought to reduce the potential for blocking antibodies and tachyphylaxis. Xeomin was introduced into the US market in 2011 and reintroduced in 2013. Its launch may be affected by the change in statistical methodology required by the FDA in reporting responder rates. Thus, the dose response curves included in the product package insert deceptively show a lower responder rate at 1 month. Using the same endpoints, however, the data would show near equivalence at 1 month. Our experience with Xeomin™ is, early comparable performance to that of Botox Cosmetic™, a similar "area of effect" with diminution of effect at 8–12 weeks using the indicated 20 units dosing in the glabella. Similar effects were seen for other indications. Botox Unit (BU) potency equivalency to Xeomin Unit (XU) is roughly 1:1.3–1:1.5. Further studies are clearly needed as the clinical trial data suggests a 1:1 ratio. Merz representatives have reported that the Xeomin vial must be inverted after reconstitution in saline to assure per bottle potency—a suggestion that some of the powder is adherent to the lid and upper surfaces of the bottle. We are aware of no published data supporting this potentially important reconstitution protocol and the Package Insert states "gently swirl" the vial. Xeomin™ is a good product and, when proper dosages are fully elucidated, could be a major player in a facial aesthetics.

What the expansion of practitioners (outside of those with core aesthetic training background) performing cosmetic treatments with NMs, there is relative lack of understanding of relevant anatomy of the facial musculature and the effects of injection (even in the upper face) that remain prevalent. Agonist–antagonist properties of the upper facial musculature must be understood for optimum outcomes. There are a paucity properly performed anatomic studies of the facial musculature that are often depicted incorrectly in anatomic diagrams [10]. This has resulted in a number of significant, albeit transient, facial deformities such as brow ptosis, eyelid hooding, "frozen" foreheads, and the "Dr. Spock" deformity. The novice practitioner is urged to focus on anatomy and dosing techniques as basic fundamental knowledge.

## Techniques by Anatomic Zone

### Glabella

Dynamic and static rhytids in the brow region are due to activity of the procerus and paired corrugator muscles. The resting tone of these muscles exerts chronic forces on the overlying skin and dermal–epidermal aging results in static rhytids. Contraction of the procerus muscle produces transverse lines at the nasion, whereas corrugator contraction results in vertical glabellar lines. Both of these features can be treated (Figs. 2.2 and 2.3) with neuromodulator injection into the glabellar area. On physical examination, the patient is asked to frown, accentuating these rhytids. The extent and course of the underlying muscles can often be visualized through the skin. Understanding the anatomy of the glabellar complex is crucial to accurate administration of the agent to achieve the desired outcome and to avoid undesirable effects (Fig. 2.4). In most individuals, the corrugator muscle is horizontally oriented, coursing along and parallel to the eyebrow. Proper treatment and dosages provide excellent clinical results with 3–6 months duration (Fig. 2.5).

The corrugator is commonly mistakenly thought to reside superior to the brow and some techniques of neuromodulator injection, including diagrams on the package insert of approved products, suggest placement of the product into this more superior position. This results in treatment of the frontalis muscle and resultant medial brow ptosis (with preserved lateral frontalis action and brow elevation), producing the "Mr. Spock" or "Mephisto" deformity (Fig. 2.6). Effective treatment of the brow, therefore, involves precise placement of the neuromodulator along the muscle belly of the corrugators, typically at the level of the brow. This can be achieved via a series of boluses throughout the muscle (author's preference) or via a threading technique (painful and inaccurate). Care must be taken to distribute the product evenly and symmetrically, unless a pre-existing asymmetry has been identified and correction is desired.

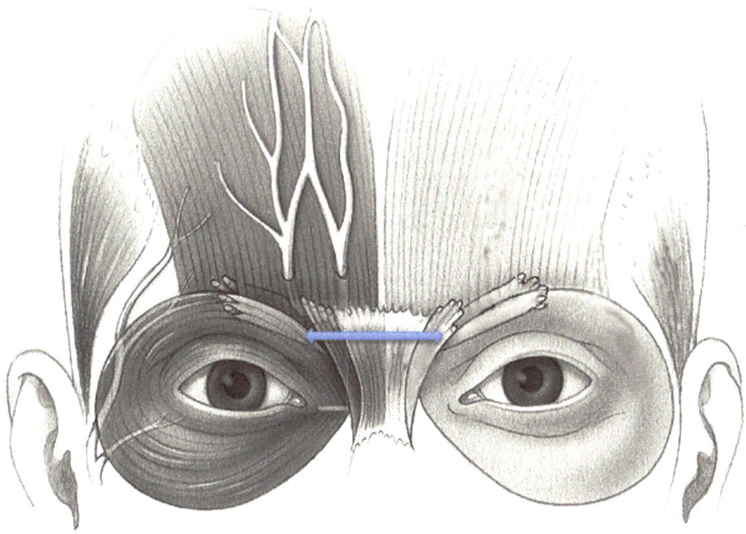

**Fig. 2.4** The corrugator supercilii courses parallel to the eyebrow and descends with the aging brow

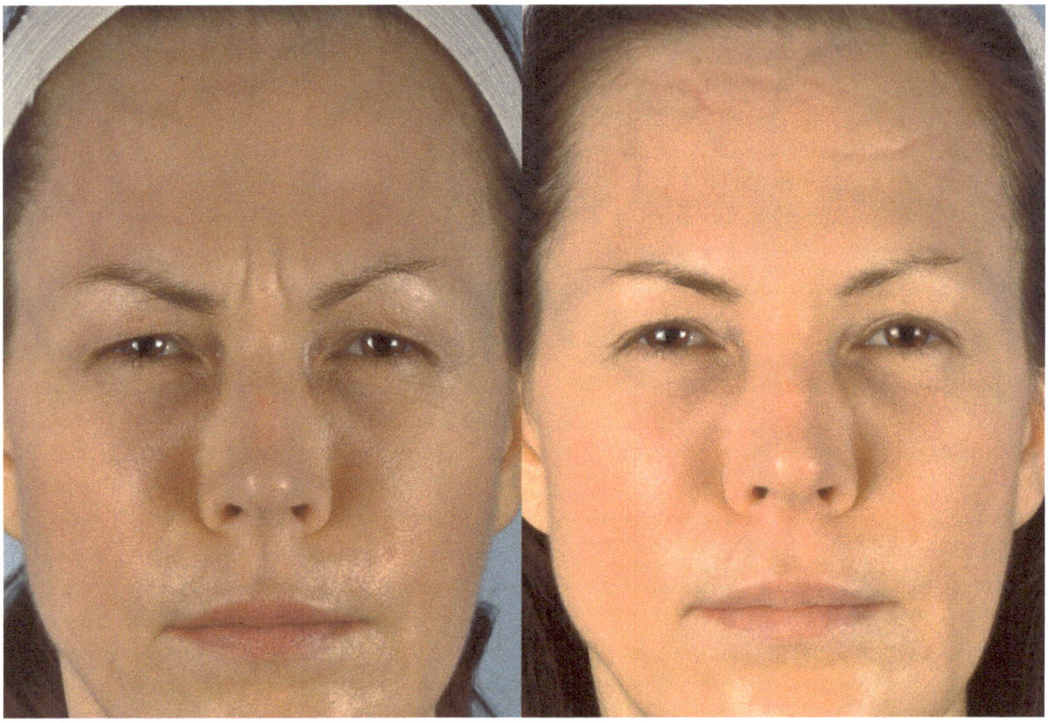

**Fig. 2.5** Xeomin glabella 30 units: before and 3 months after treatment

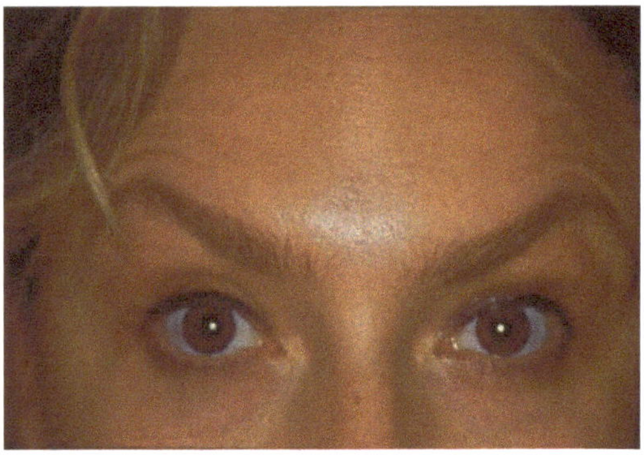

**Fig. 2.6** "Spock" or Mephisto deformity seen with glabellar injections placed too superiorly or poor distribution of frontalis injections

## Forehead

Transverse forehead rhytids are the result of frontalis activity, and neuromodulators are effective in their effacement (Fig. 2.7). The frontalis muscle exists as a continuous sheet or has a midline decussation with two muscle bellies and acts to raise the brows. Effective use of neuromodulators in the forehead requires understanding of the balance between the normal frontalis function of brow elevation and its contribution to forehead rhytids. Over-treatment of the forehead can result in undesired brow ptosis or asymmetric brows secondary to frontalis inactivation. Patients must be educated about this balance because they often present desiring total effacement of transverse forehead rhytids and this is not advisable with an understanding of the role of the frontalis in maintaining proper brow position. Physical examination should involve identification of pre-existing brow ptosis, and caution should be used in patients with this feature. In order to minimize potential brow ptosis, most patients should not be injected inferior to approximately 1.5 cm superior to the upper brow margin with limited dosages—about half of that used in the glabella and lateral orbital rhytids.

Various strategies have been used for treatment of the frontalis. The author's preference is to inject four evenly divided aliquots along the

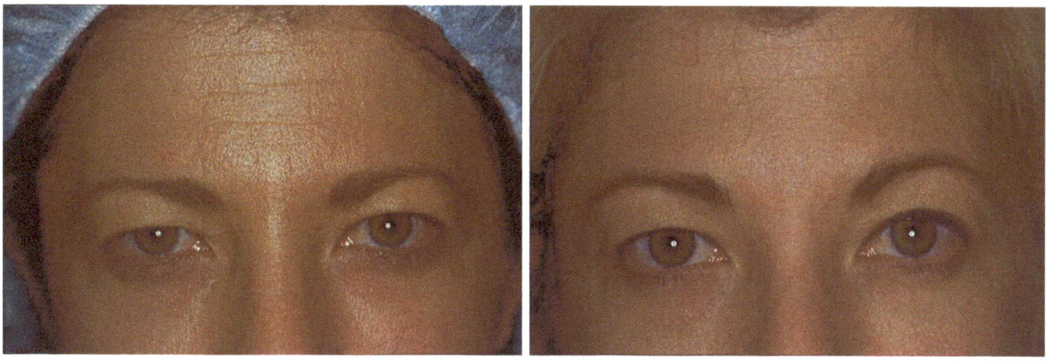

**Fig. 2.7** Forehead rhytids 10 BU. Frontalis 10 BU. Bilaterally orbicularis N.B. Brow position is maintained by releasing brow depressors

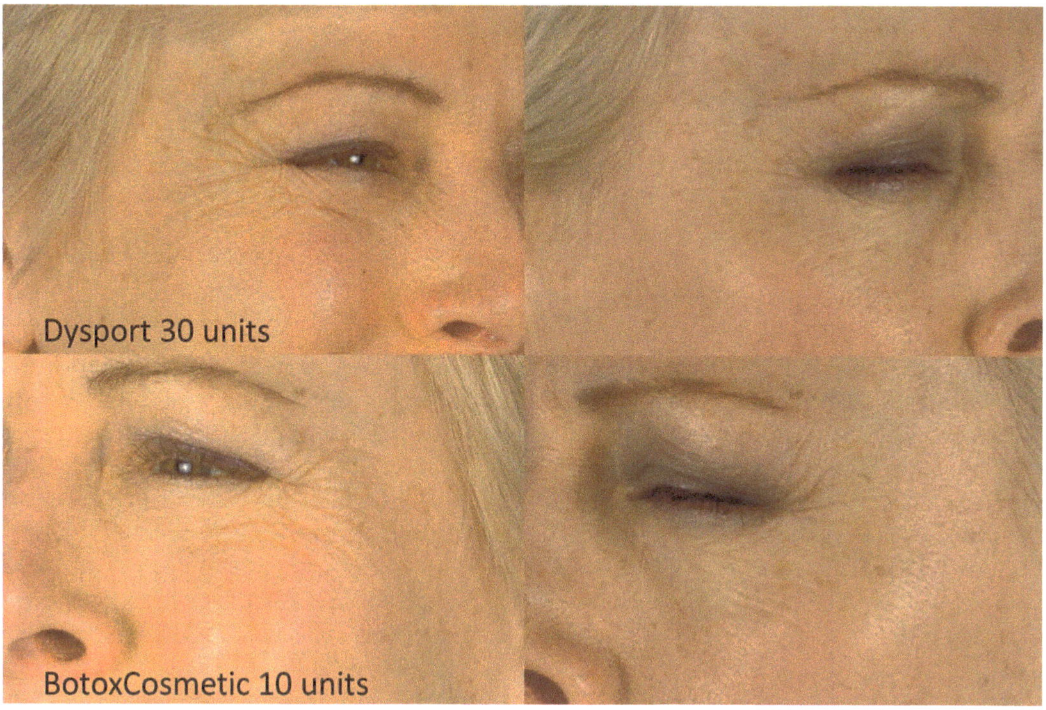


**Fig. 2.8** Lateral orbital rhytids

length of the approximately mid-forehead (Figs. 2.2 and 2.3). The medial injection point is the medial canthus, and the lateral injection point is the point at which the forehead lines curve superiorly. In patients with high forehead hairlines or rhytids that extend to or near the hairline, additional injections can be performed superiorly at the midline and between each inferior medial and lateral injection point, so as to create a zigzag injection pattern.

## Lateral Orbit

Lateral orbital rhytids or "crow's feet" are produced by the action of the orbicularis oculi muscle. This muscle functions to close the eye, pump the lacrimal system, and is also a strong brow depressor. Application of neuromodulators to the orbicularis oculi therefore alleviates crow's feet and provides some brow elevation, the latter sometimes referred to as "pharmacologic browlift" [11] (Fig. 2.8).

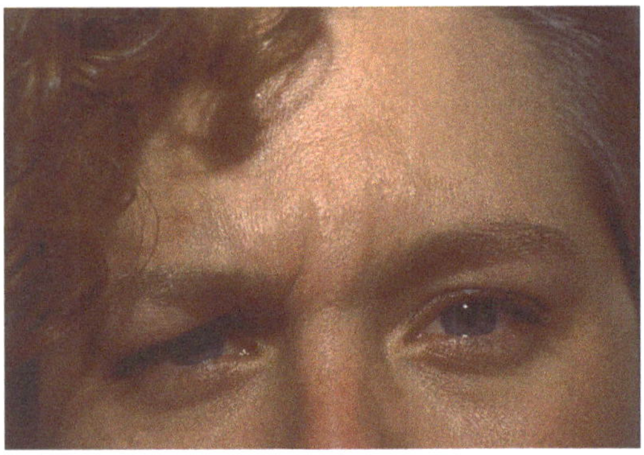

**Fig. 2.9** Patient agreed to be treated unilaterally to demonstrate the profound depressor effect of the orbicularis oculi and to a lesser extent the corrugator muscles

The orbicularis oculi muscle is located relatively superficially under the thin eyelid and periorbital skin. Effective treatment in this area involves injection of neuromodulator within the periphery of the concentric muscle, lateral to the lateral orbital rim, so as to avoid intraorbital complications and eyelid dysfunction. Care should be taken to avoid visible superficial vessels in this well-vascularized region, as needle trauma can result in significant bruising. This treatment provides a unique and marked improvement in both facial lines and brow position.

Brow position improvement is the result of reduction of the profound depressor effects of the lateral orbicularis oculi muscles as seen in Fig. 2.9. By releasing this muscle action patients can achieve up to 5 mm of brow elevation (see ref. [11]).

## Side Effects

The neuromodulators have demonstrated excellent safety and efficacy in now over 20 years of robust clinical use. The main noted side effects are local pain at the injection site, bruising, and unfavorable outcomes. Following the guidelines outlined in this chapter will provide the clinician with a lower likelihood of the latter.

One of the few transient, albeit disturbing, measurable side effects that have a measurable frequency is eyelid ptosis (Fig. 2.10). While the clinical trials showed low single digit incidences of eyelid ptosis, in practice the occurrence is quite rare (in our clinic less than 1 %). Theories as to the origin of this side effect being diffusion subcutaneously or submuscularly the full distance to the levator muscle seem unlikely. We believe that patients with supratrochlear notch (vs. foramen) are more likely to suffer this side effect.

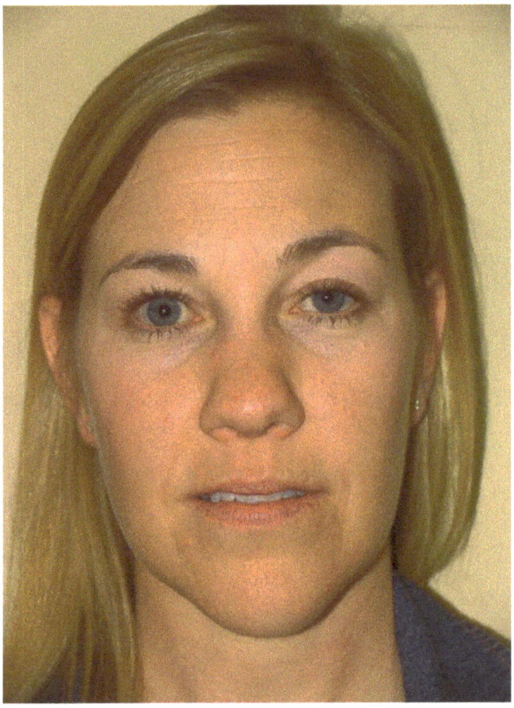

**Fig. 2.10** Eyelid ptosis. Treatment with iopidine 0.1 % eyedrops every 4–6 h as needed

Patients should be educated as to the low but measurable risk of this side effect and treatment with iopidine 0.1 % begun immediately. Reassurance is critical here as most patients will see this side effect last more than 2–3 weeks.

## Conclusions

The indications, techniques, and usage of NMs have dramatically increased over the last 10 years. Despite this expansion, many misunderstandings and myths remain about anatomy, dosage, and peritreatment care. The clinician is encouraged to pursue opinions in the literature and seek direct clinical training and updates on best practices.

## References


1. Scott AB. Botulinum toxin injection of eye muscles to correct strabismus. Trans Am Ophthalmol Soc. 1981; 79:734–70.
2. Carruthers JD, Carruthers JA. Treatment of glabellar frown lines with C. botulinum-a exotoxin. J Dermatol Surg Oncol. 1992;18(1):17–21.
3. Schantz EJ, Johnson EA. Properties and use of botulinum toxin and other microbial neurotoxins in medicine. Microbiol Rev. 1992;56(1):80–99.
4. Mosby's Medical Dictionary (8th ed. Elsevier; 2009).
5. Kim EJ, Ramirez AL, Reeck JB, Maas CS. Plast Reconstr Surg. 2003;112(5 Suppl):88S–93; discussion 94S–97.
6. Ramirez AL, Reeck J, Maas CS. Otolaryngol Head Neck Surg. 2002;126(5):459–67.
7. Dayan SH, Maas CS. Botulinum toxins for facial wrinkles: beyond glabellar lines. Facial Plast Surg Clin North Am. 2007;15(1):41–9.
8. Maas C, Kane MA, Bucay VW, Allen S, Applebaum DJ, Baumann L, Cox SE, Few JW, Joseph JH, Lorenc ZP, Moradi A, Nestor MS, Schlessinger J, Wortzman M, Lawrence I, Lin X, Nelson D. Current aesthetic use of abobotulinumtoxinA in clinical practice: an evidence-based consensus review. Aesthet Surg J. 2012;32(1 Suppl):8S–29.
9. Nettar KD, Yu KC, Bapna S, Boscardin J, Maas CS. An internally controlled, double-blind comparison of the efficacy of onabotulinumtoxinA and abobotulinumtoxinA. Arch Facial Plast Surg. 2011;13(6): 380–6.
10. Loos BM, Maas CS. Relevant anatomy for botulinum toxin facial rejuvenation. Facial Plast Surg Clin North Am. 2003;11(4):439–43.
11. Ahn MS, Catten M, Maas CS. Temporal brow lift using botulinum toxin A. Plast Reconstr Surg. 2000; 105(3):1129–35.

# Periorbital Chemical Peels

# 3

Julie A. Edween

## Abbreviations

| | |
|---|---|
| AHA | Alpha hydroxy acids |
| BHA | Beta hydroxy acids |
| BTX-A | Botulinum toxin A |
| TCA | Trichloroacetic acid |

Nonsurgical techniques for rejuvenation have seen an exponential growth with the recent advancements in technology as a response to an increase in patient demand for procedures with minimal downtime. Chemical peels are a time-tested procedure in skin rejuvenation, and despite technological growth, continue to survive as an important adjunctive procedure in the nonsurgical periocular armamentarium. Chemical peeling is the process of wounding the skin with a chemical agent, causing a controlled partial thickness burn and inflammation. The goal is to achieve in uniform exfoliation, and the stimulation new epidermal growth and evenly distributed melanin. Periorbital rhytids, photodamage, and dyschromias are reliably and predictably improved after the chemical peel.

Electronic supplementary material The online version of this chapter (doi:10.1007/978-1-4614-8388-5_3) contains supplementary material, which is available to authorized users.

J.A. Edween, D.O., F.A.O.C.O., F.A.C.S. (✉)
Facial Plastic & Cosmetic Surgery, 416 North Bedford Drive Suite 210, Beverly Hills, CA 90210, USA
e-mail: jedween@yahoo.com

## History

The use of chemical peels to beautify skin has been around since ancient times. Cleopatra used to bathe in goats' milk, whereas the women in Rome rubbed the fermented grape skins from the bottom of wine barrels to enhance their skin's beauty, unknowingly benefiting from the exfoliative properties of lactic acid [1] and tartaric acid, a common alpha hydroxy acid still used in cosmetics today [2]. The origins of the procedure in the United States are traced back to Europe, where Gypsies passed the formulas down through the ages. Chemical peels have since evolved into a procedure where guidelines, indications, and limitations have helped practitioners obtain reproducible results with improved safety and efficacy.

## Types of Chemical Peels

The chemical peel procedure involves applying chemicals to the skin to remove the outer damaged layers. This accelerates the normal process of exfoliation and results in rejuvenation of the skin. Chemical peeling of the skin of the eyelids and periorbital area results in formation of new epidermis, dermal collagen, elastin fibers, and blood vessels. This formation of new epidermis and new dermal collagen results in skin shrinkage, reduction of wrinkling and crepe paper skin, and softening of crow's feet [3].

S.A. Myint (ed.), *Nonsurgical Peri-orbital Rejuvenation*, DOI 10.1007/978-1-4614-8388-5_3,

**Table 3.1** Types of peels

| Type | Depth of penetration | Solution |
|---|---|---|
| Superficial | Epidermis | Alpha hydroxy acids:<br>20–70 % Glycolic acid, lactic, citric, tartaric<br>Beta hydroxy acids<br>20–30 % Salicylic acid<br>Lipo-hydroxy acid<br>Jessner's peel (salicylic, lactic, resorcinol)<br>10–25 % TCA |
| Medium | Papillary | 25–35 % Trichloroacetic acid<br>Trichloroacetic acid and solid $CO_2$<br>Trichloroacetic acid and Jessner's<br>Trichloroacetic acid and 70 % Glycolic<br>50 % Trichloroacetic acid |
| Deep | Reticular | Phenol |

**Table 3.2** Jessner's formula

| | |
|---|---|
| Resorcinol | 14 g |
| Salicylic acid | 14 g |
| Lactic acid | 14 mL |
| Ethanol | 100 mL |

The diversity and flexibility of chemical peels enable the physician to tailor a specific treatment for the patient. The types of chemical peels are categorized based on the various depths of penetration to the skin. Chemical peels can be divided into one of three depths: superficial, medium, and deep (Table 3.1).

## Superficial Peels

Superficial depth chemical peels are the mildest of all chemical peels and are indicated for all skin types. They are generally well tolerated and safe with rare complications. These peels create an inflammatory response from the epidermis to the stratum granulosum, or upper papillary dermis. Patients with pigmentary dyschromias, minimal photodamage, and the mildest of rhytids will benefit from superficial peels.

Alpha hydroxy acids (AHA) are extracts from fruits and vegetables and are common agents in superficial peels. Examples include glycolic acid from sugar cane, citric acid from citrus, and lactic acid from milk. The beta hydroxy acids (BHA), salicylic acid and lipo-hydroxy acid, are also agonized as superficial peels, although less commonly used. The AHA and BHA are manufactured in varying strengths and are commonly found incorporated in the many of the cosmetics and in skin maintenance cosmeceutical regimens today. Glycolic acids are one of the most frequently used alpha hydroxy acids, and in the delicate periorbital area, concentrations up to 70 % may be used with careful observation [4]. Caution should be taken when working with glycolic acid, its application is time-dependent, and a neutralizing solution such as water is used to counteract the action. These peels are extensively used today in both physician offices and by trained aestheticians.

The concentration of trichloroacetic acid (TCA) may be adjusted to create a superficial, medium, or deep peel. Low concentrations of 10–25 % generate superficial peels. Trichloroacetic acid at these concentrations produces superficial coagulation of skin proteins and destruction of the epidermis and upper papillary dermis, followed by dermal rejuvenation with new collagen deposition and normalization of elastic tissue [5]. For lower eyelid dyschromias and mild rhytidosis, 20 % TCA is an effective superficial peeling agent. Clinical indication of the depth of penetration of a TCA peel is judged by the intensity of the skin frost, with superficial peels exhibiting erythema or erythema with a light frost.

Used alone, Jessner's solution (Table 3.2) is a superficial peeling agent which acts as a keratolytic, by targeting the intracellular bridges between keratinocytes. It is depth-dependent, and the penetration used to achieve exfoliation is generally achieved using one to three chemical coats. The first clinical response after if application is mild erythema followed by a light powdery frost of the skin.

Re-epithelialization for superficial chemical peels is usually complete within a few days, with beneficial results lasting between 2 and 3 weeks.

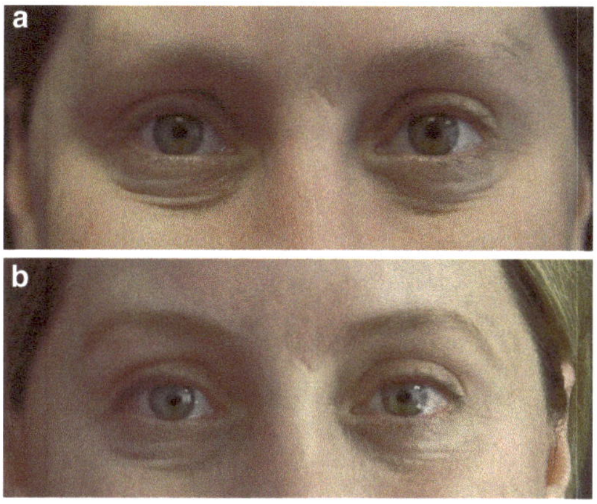


**Fig. 3.1** A 45-year-old woman before (**a**) and after (**b**) a combination Jessner's and 35 % TCA of the periorbital area. Note the reduction of dermatochalasis (excess skin) of the lower lid

Patients will notice improvement in skin texture and mild dyschromias, accompanied with a generalized brightening around the periocular area. Since the effects of superficial peels are cumulative, a series of peels repeated at regular intervals (every 4–6 weeks) may be indicated to maintain the results.

## Medium-Depth Peels

Medium-depth peels create a skin injury depth from the epidermis to the upper portions of the papillary dermis. These peels are a widespread peel of choice in the periocular region due to its uniform penetration, consistent results, and favorable risk/benefit ratio. Patients that present with crosshatched skin in the lower lid area, crow's feet, superficial rhytids, and moderate amount of sun damage often benefit from medium-depth peels (Figs. 3.1, 3.2, and 3.3).

The spectrum of medium-depth TCA concentrations starts from 30 % and generally does not exceed 50 % [6]. Concentrations of 50 % or greater have lost favor, as the results are unreliable and have been shown to greatly increase the risk of postoperative scarring [7]. Variables such as the concentration, time of application, and application technique influence the outcome of a TCA peel and are therefore vastly operator-dependent.

Over time, practitioners began combining the lower concentrations of TCA with other agents. The combination produced a deeper penetration of the wounding agent without the associated complications of higher concentrations of TCA [8]. Combinations of TCA with other agents have been described by Monheit with Jessner's solution [9], Brody and Haily [10] with solid carbon dioxide [10], and by Coleman with 70 % glycolic acid [11, 12]. The authors discovered that these combinations obtain deeper penetration of the wounding agent and have proven to be equal as the use of 50 % TCA but without its associated complications.

The combination peel described by Monheit begins with the application of Jessner's solution and then sequentially follows with the 35 % TCA. The Jessner's peel functions as an exfoliant and superficial peel, removing the stratum corneum and penetrating down to the basal layer of the epidermis, allowing for a deeper penetration of the 35 % TCA and a more even application of the peeling solution [13]. This combination Jessner's/35 % TCA peel has been shown to produce predicable results with a measured decrease in complications. Patients generally develop a light crusting in 3–5 days and will exfoliate completely in 7–10 days. Patients may return back to work in 7 days, using light makeup to cover the pink and erythematous color of the freshly peeled skin. This combination medium-depth peel is the author's peel of choice in the periorbital area and will be described in detail in this chapter.

TCA solutions are prepared commercially or in the office from crystals mixed with distilled water and compounded in a weight-to-volume preparation. Clear communication with those preparing the solution is paramount, bringing attention to the fact that the dilution is weight to volume, assuring a standardized concentration. The solution should be carefully mixed before usage due to potential settling of crystals. It is stable at room temperature and not light-sensitive, but care must be taken to make sure the bottles are closed securely, as evaporation will increase the concentration of the solution.

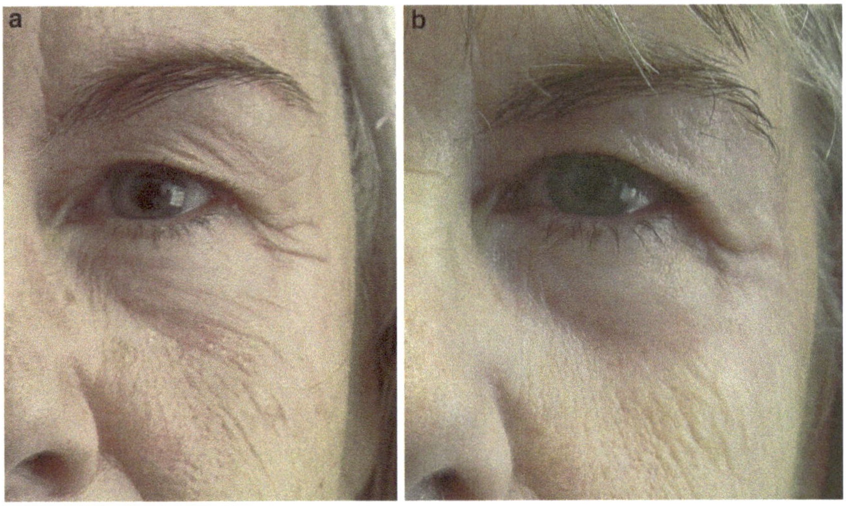

**Fig. 3.2** A 50-year-old woman before (**a**) and after (**b**) a combination of Jessner's and 35 % TCA of the periorbital area. An improvement of the dyschromias and wrinkling is evident

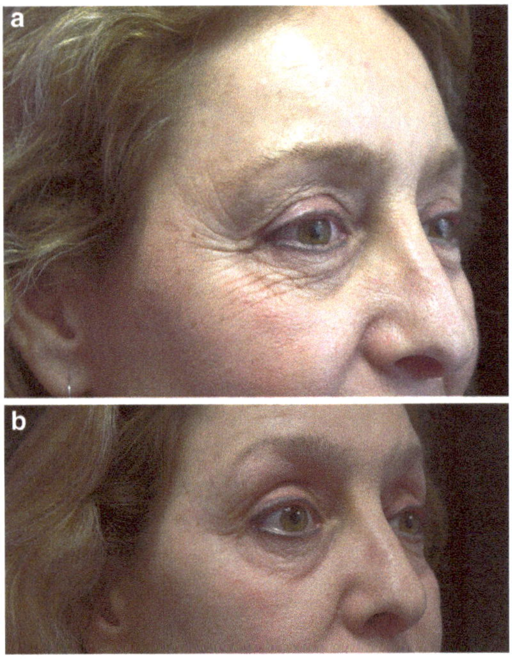

**Fig. 3.3** A 49-year-old woman before (**a**) and after (**b**) a combination of Jessner's and 35 % TCA of the periorbital area. The crosshatched skin and rhytids in the lower lid area show overall improvement

## Deep Chemical Peels

Deep chemical peels use chemoexfoliants that penetrate from the epidermis to the mid reticular dermis. They effectively resurface deeper periocular rhytids, crepey appearance, crow's feet, and severe actinic keratosis (Fig. 3.4). The Baker–Gordon formula (Table 3.3) is the often referenced classic deep peel and has given rise to various authors developing modifications of the phenol–croton oil-based formula. The reaction following application of the phenol is characterized by keratocoagulative necrosis of the epidermis extending into the papillary dermis and by a marked inflammatory reaction [14]. The healing process takes place over 8–14 days with post-peel redness continuing up to 2 months [15]. The lasting and restorative effects make phenol peeling ideal for patients seeking improvement of deeper rhytids and creases in the periorbital area.

Because of the depth of the wounding of the skin, these peels have a prolonged healing time and higher risk of complications such as hypopigmentation and scarring. Discretion should be used in patients with a history of hepatic, cardiac, and renal disease, as it can affect hepatic and renal function and has reportedly caused suppression of pulmonary function and cardiac activity [16]. Phenol is directly toxic to the myocardium, necessitating the need for full cardiopulmonary monitoring. To minimize these complications, the solution is applied slowly and systematically to individual aesthetic units over a prescribed period of time, while monitoring carefully for cardiac arrhythmias before proceeding to the

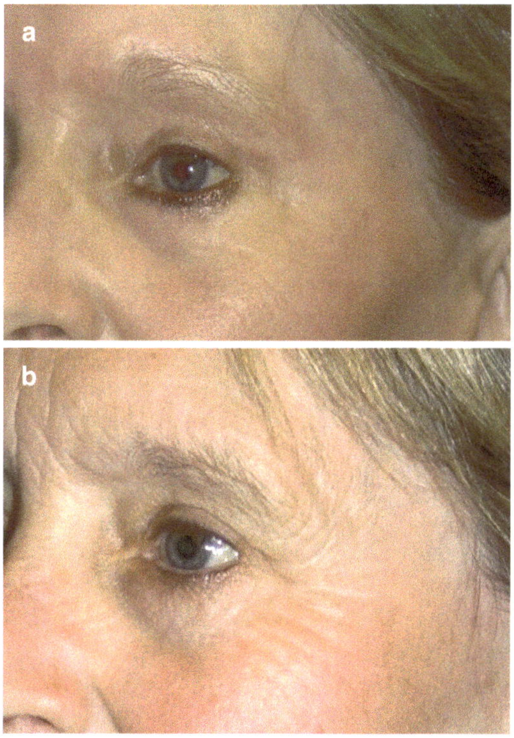

**Fig. 3.4** A 70-year-old woman before (**a**) and after (**b**) a phenol peel of the periorbital area. She has had a previous blepharoplasty. Note the dramatic resolution of the periorbital rhytids and wrinkles

**Table 3.3** The Baker–Gordon formula

| |
|---|
| 3 mL 89 % Liquid phenol (USP) |
| 2 mL Tap water |
| Eight drops of liquid soap (Septisol) |
| Three drops of croton oil |

next subunit. These peels have a considerable learning curve and should be reserved for physicians with a comprehensive understanding of complexity of peels and considerable level of experience with the procedure.

## Patient Selection

### Indications

Proper patient selection is paramount for successful outcomes. The physician should customize the procedure with the patient's goals, establish patient compliance, and manage expectations.

**Table 3.4** Fitzpatrick classification scale

| Skin type | Skin color | Characteristics |
|---|---|---|
| I | White; very fair, red/blond hair; blue eyes, freckles | Always burns, never tans |
| II | White; very fair, red/blond hair; blue, hazel, or green eyes | Usually burns, tans with difficulty |
| III | Cream white; fair with any hair or eye color; very common | Sometimes mild burn, gradually tans |
| IV | Brown; typical Mediterranean Caucasian skin | Rarely burns, tans with ease |
| V | Dark brown; Middle Eastern skin types | Very rarely burns, tans very easily |
| VI | Black | Never burns, tans very easily |

Patient assessment begins with the evaluation of skin type, severity of rhytids, amount of redundant skin, degree of laxity of the lower eyelid margin, thickness of the dermal skin around the eyes, actinic damage, and dyschromias. Clarifying the difference between rhytids due to sun damage from that of volume loss and need for a blepharoplasty is necessary for both the patient and physician to recognize.

The Fitzpatrick skin color classification (Table 3.4) is a convenient means in evaluating skin color type and its reaction to sun exposure. Once skin type is identified, the Glogau classification system (Table 3.5), which assesses skin texture, skin thickness, degree of photodamage, and severity of wrinkles, will guide in choosing the appropriate peel. In conjunction with a patient's medical history and lifestyle, the physician will be able to further tailor the treatment for the patient condition.

Superficial peels are effective for Fitzpatrick skin types I–V and Glogau I patients with mild sun damage and fine wrinkling around the eye area. Sometimes referred to as "refresher" peels, these peels may require repeat treatments to maintain desired results.

The medium-depth peel provides a safe resurfacing modality for moderate photoaging and rhytids (Glogau II) and Fitzpatrick skin types I–IV. Peeling higher Fitzpatrick skin types should be guarded and performed only by experienced practitioners, as Kadhim reports fine and medium periorbital wrinkles responded favorably with

**Table 3.5** The Glogau classification scale

| Skin class | Description |
|---|---|
| I | Early wrinkles<br>Age: Twenties to thirties<br>Early photoaging<br>Mild pigment changes<br>Minimal wrinkles<br>No "age spots" |
| II | Wrinkles in motion<br>Age: Thirties to forties<br>Early to moderate photoaging<br>Appearance of smile lines<br>Early brown "age spots"<br>Early changes in skin texture |
| III | Wrinkles at rest<br>Age: Fifties and older<br>Advanced photoaging<br>Prominent brown pigmentation<br>Visible brown "age spots"<br>Small blood vessels<br>Wrinkles, even at rest |
| IV | Only wrinkles<br>Age: Sixties and older<br>Severe photoaging<br>Yellow-gray skin color<br>Prior skin cancers<br>Precancerous skin changes (actinic keratosis) |

medium-depth chemical peels with low and mild adverse effects in dark-skinned individuals [17].

Deeper, coarse rhytids and marked photoaging respond effectively to deeper peels with resultant dramatic and long-lasting effects. The optimum candidate is a Glogau III and IV and a Fitzpatrick I and II and generally not considered for darker skin types due to a high incidence of hypopigmentation.

## History

The Patients' thorough medical and drug history must be throughly evaluated. Relative contraindications for any resurfacing procedure include cutaneous radiation history, active or frequent herpes simplex virus infections, diabetes, hypertrophic scar, or keloid history [18].

Previous history of isotretinoin (Accutane, Roche, Nutley, NJ) usage is a relative contraindication, as the scaring that may result after a peel can be devastating. Isotretinoin prevents post-peel reepithelialization, and a cessation period of 12–24 months is recommended prior to the peel [18].

Birth control pills, exogenous estrogens (soaps, creams, oils), or photosensitizing drugs are to be avoided due to the risk of hyperpigmentation. Because of the level of estrogen in pregnancy, the patient should avoid plans to become pregnant within the first 6 months of the peel [19].

Patients with a history of herpes simplex require antiviral prophylaxis prior to the peel and continued after until re-epithelialization is complete. Antiviral treatment regimens such as valacyclovir (Valtrex, Glaxo Wellcome, West Caldwell, NJ) 500 mg twice a day 2 days prior to the peel, followed by 5 days after the peel, are prescribed. This treatment averts most herpetic breakouts during the post-healing process. Alternative antiviral regimens exist and some physicians advocate prophylactic antivirals to all patients undergoing the peel.

If the patient has had a previous blepharoplasty, or a previous peel, check the ability for the upper lid to completely close. If the upper lid does not fully close, peeling of the upper eyelid is contraindicated due to the potential upper lid tightening, incomplete lid closure, and resultant globe desiccation.

## Lifestyle

For a patient to qualify for the peeling procedure, it is essential to examine their lifestyle and habits. They must be reliable to comply with pre- and posttreatment instructions and motivated to care for the area to ensure success of the peel. A prescreening questionnaire reviewing the patient's daily activities, occupation, and hobbies will identify areas of concern.

Smoking is a relative contraindication and smokers should agree to stop 1 month prior to peel and continue for at least 6 weeks after. Patients that have frequent sun exposure need to commit to making a lifestyle change that involves sun avoidance and protecting the area from the sun. Patient acceptance and agreement with peel protocols are paramount in avoiding complications. If there is any doubt regarding their compliance, they should be disqualified from being treated with a peel.

## Pretreatment Preparation

Proper preparation of patient and skin is mandatory to achieve consistent, reliable results and to prevent post-procedure complications.

The author treats almost all patients with a combination of topical 0.05 % tretinoin (Retin-A Ortho Pharmaceutical, Raritan, NJ) and hydroquinone 4 % for at least 4 weeks and up to 6 weeks prior to peel. This regimen decreases the stratum corneum thickness, provides an even chemical uptake, and allows better epithelial regeneration and dermal fibroblast activity, for a more rapid post-procedural healing process [20, 21]. The use of hydroquinone, which suppresses melanocyte activity, aids in preventing postinflammatory hyperpigmentation that can occur following epidermal injury from peeling agents. Adequate pretreatment of the skin facilitates a more uniform response of the penetration of the peel, leading to a more consistent result. Patients are instructed to follow an application schedule of tretinoin and hydroquinone twice a week for the first week, followed by three times a week, every other day, and up to every day as tolerated. Some redness and minor skin irritation is expected; however, adjustments to the application interval and dosage may be necessary if the patient develops retinoid dermatitis. If retinoid dermatitis is present, then it is advisable to wait at least 1 week before performing the peeling procedure.

Patients are instructed to avoid frequent exposure to the sun, wear sunscreen, and abstain from waxing, dermabrasion, electrolysis, and lasers for 3–4 weeks prior to peeling [18].

Informed consents are signed by all patients prior to peeling, which acknowledges the possibility of scarring, infection, prolonged erythema, pigmentary changes, and pain at minimum. It is beneficial for patients to gain a clear understanding of the peeling process by preparing patients of expected events during and after the peeling procedure. Photographs are taken before and after the procedure to document changes and also serve as a reminder for the patient that may not recollect their former skin presentation.

## Procedure of Combination Jessner's and 35 % TCA Medium-Depth Peel

Preoperative anesthesia varies with the individual physician's preference, the depth of the peel to be applied, and the patient's own anxiety level. Most patients do quite well throughout the procedure with a single dose of 0.5 mg alprazolam (Xanax, Pfizer, New York, NY) given 30 min prior to the peel. While additional anesthesia is not necessary, patients with higher anxiety levels can benefit from using regional nerve blocks, 1 % lidocaine, to the supraorbital, infraorbital, zygomaticofrontal, and zygomaticotemporal nerves. A handheld fan is also provided to help reduce the discomfort during the application of the peel.

The physician should be standing at the head of the table and lean over the patient so the physician and patient are face to face. The patient is placed in a seated position, preferably at a 45-degree angle.

Safety precautions are important to insure efficient peel. The solutions are placed in order of usage from left to right in clearly labeled surgical cups. Our setup from left to right consists of acetone, Jessner's solution, and 35 % trichloroacetic acid. A 2×2 gauze is placed in front of the acetone solution and cotton-tipped applicators are placed in a single cup and thrown away after each use (Fig. 3.5).

The patient is requested to cleanse their skin the night before and the morning of the procedure. They are instructed not to use any makeup

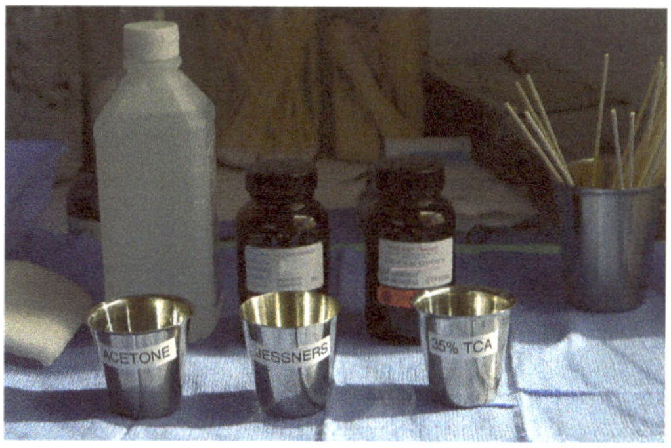


**Fig. 3.5** Setup for a combination Jessner's and 35 % trichloroacetic acid medium-depth peel

or apply moisturizers or sunscreen on the day of the procedure. All patients will additionally cleanse with Cetaphil (Galderma Labs, Fort Worth, TX) upon arrival to the office. Thoroughly cleansed skin is crucial to obtain uniform uptake of the peel.

The patient's skin is first gently degreased with wrung out 2×2 gauze soaked in acetone applied to the upper and lower eyelid area in a uniform fashion. A small handheld fan can be used to diffuse the fumes from the acetone. Prior degreasing removes surface skin oils and residual makeup, allowing the chemical to have the best contact with the stratum corneum. Inadequate degreasing may result in an uneven penetration and produce varying levels of peel.

To protect the globe from any possible damage from accidental chemical leaking into the eye, a sterile ophthalmic ointment Lacri-lube (Allergan, Inc., Irvine, CA) is used to act as a physical barrier before the procedure. An assistant stands present to promptly blot any tears, as tears can channel and pull the chemical into the eye by capillary action, causing a corneal burn. Eyewash solution such as balanced salt solution is readily available in case of accidental exposure. In the event of this occurrence, the eye should be immediately flushed with the solution, followed by placing an antibiotic/steroid ointment into the eye and referred for an ophthalmologic consult.

The Jessner's solution is applied first and spread with a cotton-tipped applicator, with the excess rolled out against the side of the cup. This allows the precise application of the solution and avoids any excess. A uniform wetness to the applicator is encouraged, as the wetter the applicator, the deeper the depth of penetration. The solution is then spread without using force. On the first application pass, inform the patient they may experience a painful burning sensation and remind them to use the handheld fan to control discomfort if necessary. The discomfort may provoke tearing. Have your assistant ready with a cotton-tipped applicator to promptly dab away the tears to avoid contact with the peeled areas.

A standard sequential pattern is followed when applying the chemical to the individual periocular subunits. The subunits of the eye are divided into the lateral crow's feet, infrabrow area, upper eyelid, and lower eyelid. The physician begins on one periocular subunit, followed by contralateral subunit of the opposite eye. For example, start by applying the solution to the right lateral crow's feet, followed by the left lateral crow's feet. By doing so it allows the physician to better reproduce the depth and frost of the treatment and assures that areas are not skipped. The author begins in the upper eyelid region while the patients eyes are closed, using the application sequence pattern described by Morrow [3]. The solution is applied to the crow's feet area first, superior to the lateral canthal angle, proceeding medially along the inferior border of the eyebrow, then inferiorly down to the eyelash margin, the inner canthus, and root of the nose. Applying the solution into the eyebrow area is safe and the eyebrow cilia are unharmed during the process. For the lower lid complex, the solution is applied with the eyes open, looking superiorly. Patients are instructed that they may blink all they want, but they have to keep their eyes open. The solution is applied from the lateral malar and orbital rim, across the crow's feet, moving superiorly and medially to the eyelash margin. When first gaining familiarity with chemical peels, it is advisable for the practitioner to adapt a more conservative approach of applying the solution no closer than 2–3 mm from the eyelash margin as described by McCollough and Hillman [22], and as one becomes more adept, progress to applying up to the eyelash margin, as safely demonstrated by Morrow [3].

The Jessner's solution will first turn the skin pink, followed by a light frost. This frost is the endpoint and an indication of penetration through the epidermis (Fig. 3.6). After the Jessner's solution has dried, the 35 % trichloroacetic acid peel is applied with a similar sequential aesthetic subunit technique, using rolled out cotton-tipped applicators. Thicker skin of the crow's feet, infrabrow, and upper and lower eyelids can tolerate a stronger application with one to two cotton-tipped applicators. Patients will experience an intense burning sensation; again remind the patient that they may use their fan for their cooling

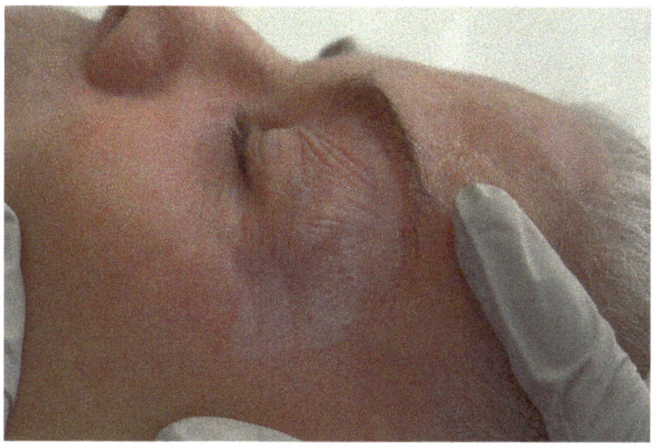

**Fig. 3.6** Application of the Jessner's peel. The skin will turn slight pink with a light frost. It is the clinical endpoint of the peel's penetration into the epidermis

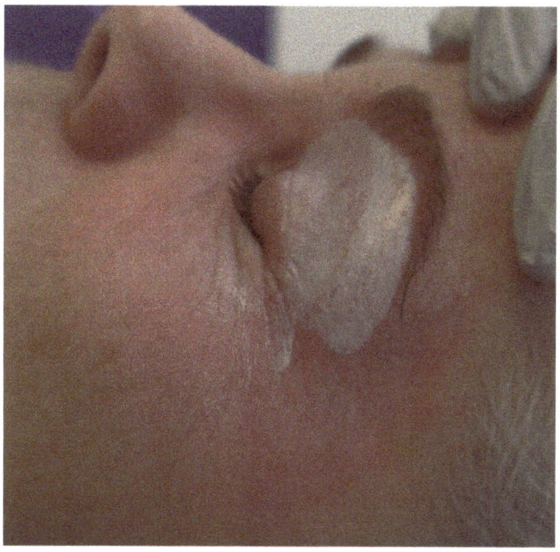

**Fig. 3.7** Application of the 35 % trichloroacetic acid peel. Note the solid white background, the clinical indication that the wounding solution has penetrated into the papillary dermis

comfort. The delicate thin skin of the inner canthus and tarsal plates requires lighter pressure. Make sure the cotton-tipped applicator is rolled out well, applied lightly, and almost "feathered" in this area. Feathering techniques are used for fair-skinned patients with considerable sun exposure, since it aids in blending the line of demarcation between the areas of peeled and non-peeled.

For fine to medium rhytids around the periorbital area, applying the 35 % trichloroacetic acid with broad strokes is effective. Modifications may be made during the peeling process since areas may show decreased uptake of solution and call for additional passes. For deeper rhytids, the skin can be stretched out to assure contact and uniform penetration of the solution into the deep creases, and the wooden end of a cotton-tipped applicator can be used for precise application of the chemical solution until desired endpoint is achieved.

After the first application pass of the 35 % TCA, wait approximately 3–4 min for the frosting to peak assess the quality of the peeled area for needed repeat applications [8]. Areas of patchy or uneven frosting should be retreated carefully with a thin application of TCA. A thick uniform white frost indicates the application endpoint (Fig. 3.7). Once the frost has dissipated and the skin is pink, an occlusive ointment such as Aquaphor (Eucerin, Brookfield, CT) is sparingly applied to prevent desiccation. Upon completion of the peel, patients may continue to experience an acute burning sensation, lasting for approximately 30 min to an hour. To alleviate the burning sensation, a 2 × 2 gauze dipped in ice water placed on area can provide immediate symptomatic relief.

## Depth of Peel

The physician must decide what depth of penetration is necessary to produce the desired outcome. The level of penetration of a peel is influenced by several factors such as:

The type of peeling agent
Concentration of peeling agent
Number of passes applied
Duration of time in contact with skin
Wetness of the applications
Pressure used in application (vigorous rubbing vs. light painting strokes)
Pretreatment to prime skin
The type of skin and its condition

Understanding the properties of the chosen chemical agent is important in using them successfully. Generally, the whiter the frost, the deeper into the dermis the TCA has penetrated (Table 3.6). The white color or "frost" from TCA appears as a consequence of epidermal and der-

**Table 3.6** Depth of peel

| | |
|---|---|
| Superficial | Erythema with stringy or light frost |
| Medium | White coat with slight background erythema |
| Deep | Solid opaque white with minimal or no background erythema |

mal protein coagulation [12]. Superficial TCA peels in concentrations of 10–25 % are indicated for superficial rhytids on most skin types with minimal recovery time and rare complications. TCA applied in light concentrations manifests as an erythematous appearance with a light frost, indicating penetration into the papillary dermis and coagulation of epidermal proteins. With an increase in concentration of the peeling solution, the frost becomes more uniform, and a distinct white color becomes apparent. Medium-depth peels such as the combination Jessner's and 35 % TCA peel targets moderate rhytids that extend to the upper reticular dermis, with the clinical indicator of a distinct white frost with slight erythema showing through appearing in about 5–10 min. This distinct white frost is a transient phenomenon and the skin will then rebound with perfusion, and capillary refill should be present within 20 min [8]. For deep peels such as 50 % TCA, the endpoint is a dense uniform white frost that dissipates in 40–50 min [12]. If the peeling solution penetrates the deep dermis, the skin will have a grayish white hue. This is not desirable, indicating destruction to the dermis, resulting in late healing and possible hypertrophic scarring.

## Postoperative Considerations

Patients are informed to expect edema, erythema, and desquamation in the healing process. The use of ice water compresses (2×2 nonsterile gauze, soaked in ice water, and wrung out gently) will serve to minimize swelling and provide symptomatic relief from burning during the initial 24 h. It is suggested that patients sleep with their head elevated to offset the edema around the eyelids, which at times may prevent the eyelids from opening. On the morning after the procedure, the patient should start cleansing with a mild cleanser such as Cetaphil (Galderma Labs, Fort Worth, TX) twice a day, followed by the application of Aquaphor ointment.

Erythema of the skin, followed by tightening, swelling, and a gradual skin color change to dark brown and gray, is to be expected. The skin should then start to slough by the third to fourth post-procedure day. After the skin begins to peel, patients are instructed to soak the area twice a day with wrung out 0.25 % acetic acid soaks made of one tablespoon in one pint of warm water. After the soaks, a thin coat of petrolatum jelly or Aquaphor (Beiersdorf Inc., Hamburg, Germany) is placed on the skin, which prevents desiccation and promotes re-epithelialization. The patient is advised not to pick or actively peel away any dark skin during the desquamation process. After the skin shed is complete, traditionally around 4–5 days, the skin will re-epithelialize and appear bright pink in about a week and slowly fade to a natural skin color over the following 3 weeks. Note that when the upper and lower eyelids are peeled, the upper eyelids may heal a few days slower than the lower eyelids due to the continued movement of the upper eyelid skin at the crease, delaying re-epithelialization. After the peeling is complete, the patient can use a light oil-free moisturizer and makeup can be used to cover the area.

Avoiding the sun is imperative and patients are advised to wear wrap around UV protective filtering sunglasses and as well as a wide-brimmed hat when outdoors. Photoprotection with a broad spectrum sunscreen SPF 30 can be used when re-epithelialization is complete and continued for at least 6 weeks to minimize the risk of developing hyperpigmentation. In patients with sensitive skin, it may be necessary to delay the use of sunscreen for at least a month to reduce the possibility of contact dermatitis.

A return to normal activity is expected approximately 7–10 days following the peel. When peeling is complete and significant inflammation has resolved, patients are instructed to resume the application of Retin-A. The use of Retin-A will help heal the skin faster, reduce pigmentary changes, superficial wrinkling, and smooth textural changes of the skin. Darker skin types such as Fitzpatrick III and IV are more prone to postinflammatory hyperpigmentation. If present, then a bleaching agent such as 4 % hydroquinone can be started and then tapered in usage when the pigmentation subsides.

## Complications

When first gaining experience in performing chemical peels, it is advisable to become fully familiar with superficial peels and its effects on the skin and then gradually increase to deeper peels as one gains more experience with the procedure.

### Prolonged Erythema

The deeper the wounding from the chemical peel, the longer the expected erythema. For superficial peels the erythema may last for 7–10 days, medium-depth peel 2–4 weeks, and deep peels can last months and slowly dissipate without treatment. Persistent erythema lasting for over 3 months [12] should be a warning sign for the potential development of scarring. Topical hydrocortisone 2.5 % lotion or other nonfluorinated steroid cream may be helpful in reducing the inflammatory response and thus improving the skin's appearance. Fluorinated steroid creams may lead to skin atrophy and hypopigmentation and should not be used. Oral antihistamines, short-term systemic steroids, silicone gel sheeting, and the application of a green foundation under base makeup [23] can be used to blend area until the erythema gradually fades away.

### Hyperpigmentation

Although postinflammatory hyperpigmentation is most commonly seen in darker skin types, all skin types are at risk since the process chemoexfoliation causes inflammation. Hyperpigmentation can appear patchy or as a dark brownish mask. Patches of hyperpigmentation can occur with exposure to both UV-A and UV-B light in pigment-prone individuals as well as patients who are pregnant or who are taking birth control pills, exogenous estrogens, or photosensitizing drugs [16]. During the early stages of healing, patients are instructed to practice strict sun avoidance by protecting the area with UV filtering sunglasses and to wear a wide-brimmed hat. The use of an SPF 30 sunscreen is recommended upon re-epithelialization of the skin, which generally occurs within 7–10 days. In most patients who develop hyperpigmentation, noncompliance with sun avoidance is the most common cause. If an increase in pigmentation is observed, it can frequently be stopped through application of tretinoin 0.05 and 4 % hydroquinone cream combination for a few weeks; however, it may take up to several months for hyperpigmentation to resolve.

### Hypopigmentation

As mentioned previously, preoperative evaluation of skin type and peel choice is important to control this occurrence. The deeper the peel, the more marked the contrast between the peeled and non-peeled areas. Medium-depth peels such as the Jessner's/35 % TCA cause minimal hypopigmentation. Hypopigmentation is most commonly seen in deeper peels such as 50 % trichloroacetic acid or phenol peel and with deeper wounding techniques such as vigorous rubbing of solution into skin or multiple application passes. Since phenol acts by reducing the ability of melanocytes to produce melanin, post-peel hypopigmentation is common and every patient should be informed of the expected outcome. If hypopigmentation occurs in lighter skin types Fitzpatrick I–III, it can be readily camouflaged with light makeup application. Darker skin types, Fitzpatrick IV–V, are at a greater risk, and these patients must be informed of potential permanent hypopigmentation prior to peeling at these depths. Furthermore, with darker skin types and in those patients that tan excessively, the line of demarcation may be visualized between peeled and non-peeled areas. Applying the solution lightly with a "feathering" technique will help blend this post-peel demarcation.

## Infection

Infection is prevented by judicious post-procedural skin care. Patients are instructed to follow a strict skin care regimen, which accelerates skin slough and removal of devitalized tissue in a timely fashion. Routine antibiotics for superficial and medium-depth periorbital peels are unnecessary, although some practitioners routinely use them with deep peels. The application of 0.25 % acetic acid soaks to the post-procedural skin care routine is effective as it has antibacterial properties and dissolves and cleanses devitalized tissue. The most common bacterial agent is Staphylococcus aureus, which responds well to a topical antibiotic ointment. In fact, after desquamation, some practitioners routinely employ bacitracin ointment over a petrolatum-based ointment for its antibiotic properties.

Patients with a history of herpes are pretreated with prophylactic antivirals, making outbreaks quite rare. Outbreaks will manifest with fever, pain, and vesicles in the area. If an additional outbreak manifests while patient is currently on an antiviral course, then a second antiviral may be added to the regimen with continued reassurance given throughout the healing process.

## Scarring

Scarring is least likely to occur after a superficial peel since the dermis is rarely penetrated. There is about a 1 % risk of scarring in the combination medium-depth peels (Jessner's/35 % TCA) [10], with the incidence increasing with deeper peels. Hypertrophic and elevated areas may respond favorably to biweekly injections of 0.2–0.3 mg of intralesional triamcinolone 10 mg/mL, placed in a horizontal line just inferior to the lower eyelash margin [3]. Topical silicone gels and nonfluorinated steroids are also effective.

## Cicatricial Ectropion

Careful selection of the appropriate peel for the amount of lower lid laxity is paramount in preventing excessive skin contracture during wound healing. Chemical peels cause vertical and horizontal shortening of the skin; if more shortening than is desirable occurs, it manifests as lagophthalmos with corneal exposure, lower eyelid retraction, or early lower eyelid margin ectropion or frank ectropion [24]. This area can be managed with intralesional triamcinolone, in the same manner described above for scarring. Sterile gauze strips (steri-strips) positioned from the lower lid to the upper brow, in a similar fashion as managing a postsurgical eyelid retraction, will assist in supporting the lower lid.

## Ocular Damage

To avoid spilling wounding agents, never move the applicator or brush directly over the eye area. Chemical peels may accidently reach the cornea or sclera of the eye during the application of a peel. Tear production can act as a wick when in contact with the peel and drag the chemical solution into the eye. This action can produce a burn, and if the sclera is affected, a whitish-gray color over the exposed area may be visualized. In that event, the eye should be immediately copiously irrigated with sterile saline solution; an antibiotic/steroid ointment should be placed and followed by an immediate ophthalmologic consult.

## Milia

Milia, or tiny epidermal inclusion cysts, can appear as small whiteheads on the eyelid skin after the peel. These are usually self-limited and clear with appropriate skin care. Typically they do not appear until 2–3 weeks after re-epithelialization and may be aggravated by thick ointments that occlude the upper pilosebaceous units [25]. At times it may be necessary to unroof persistent milia with an 18 gauge needle or the tip of an 11 blade scalpel.

## Chemical Peel and Blepharoplasty

Transconjunctival blepharoplasty is a reliable technique for rejuvenation of the lower lid area. It successfully removes periorbital fat, but limitations occur in addressing excessive skin and lower eyelid wrinkling. In these cases the chemical peel serves as a viable adjunctive procedure to improve the lower lid skin appearance. Periorbital chemical peels may be performed before a blepharoplasty, during surgery, or after a blepharoplasty.

Combining a transconjunctival blepharoplasty with a chemical peel provides an ideal rejuvenation to the periorbital area. It is generally safe since the skin muscle flaps have not been elevated and vascular supply is intact and not adversely altered. Superficial and medium and deep peels can be safely performed in conjunction with a transconjunctival blepharoplasty with minimal effect to the healing time. Dodenhoff has safely performed both 35 % TCA combination peel immediately following a transconjunctival blepharoplasty and also observed marked shrinkage of skin in the lower lid skin when using phenol peel [26]. Similar results with a phenol peel are described by McKinney and Zukowski who reported successful results performing a phenol peel immediately following a transconjunctival blepharoplasty [27]. When a deeper phenol peel is performed following a transconjunctival blepharoplasty, the risk of lower eyelid ectropion is higher. To minimize this complication to a minimum, caution should be exercised in individuals with subclinical or partial ectropion and minimal loss of apposition of the lid to the sclera [23].

After a transconjunctival approach, Morrow advocates peeling both the upper and lower eyelids with a 35 % trichloroacetic acid 7 days after surgery, a trichloroacetic acid 50 % or phenol 89 % after 10–14 days after surgery, and Bakers phenol peel 30 days after. With this timetable Morrow reportedly not had any complications [3]. Gatti presents the phenol peeling procedure as a secondary part of a routine lower blepharoplasty and performs the adjunctive chemical peel a minimum of 6 weeks after blepharoplasty [28]. Litton and Trinidad wait at least 6 months before proceeding with a phenol 50 % chemical peel to the eyelids [29].

When applying a chemical peel immediately following a blepharoplasty, it is vital to apply the solution with featherlike strokes in the pretarsal area and precisely stop within 1–2 mm of the fresh incision. The same precautions are taken when performed in conjunction with a lateral canthal procedure, avoiding the suture line in a similar fashion. The rest of the peel and depth of wounding is applied in the same manner as if the procedure was being performed without a blepharoplasty [26]. Thc benefit of waiting to peel after the blepharoplasty has healed is that the chemical solution can be applied directly over the old incision, aiding in lightening of the scar. Some authors recommend avoiding a lower eyelid scar altogether by endorsing the peel as a standalone procedure for the excess lower lid skin.

## Chemical Peel and Blepharoplasty

Since periorbital rhytids result from both photoaging and the repetitive contraction of the orbicularis oculi muscles [30], the combination of chemical peels with injectables comes as a sensible solution for overall rejuvenation of the periorbital area. Regarding botulinum toxin A, discussion on the appropriate timing of injection in relation to healing from the peel is ongoing. The authors experience is similar to Landau's, where BTX-A injections where successfully performed prior to and immediately after the a superficial and medium-depth peel with no excessive rate of side effects related to unexpected diffusion to remote muscles [15]. Moreover in regard to dermal fillers, Landau recommends that permanent fillers are not affected by the peeling procedure and temporary fillers are more easily absorbed because of the inflammation induced by the chemical agent and thus should be injected at least 2 weeks after the peel.

## Conclusion

Chemical peels are a time-tested tool in the nonsurgical armamentarium and very effective for rhytids and photodamage in the periorbital area. Various formulations and varieties of chemical peels exist, and the diversity makes it possible for the physician to tailor the treatment to the desired outcome. Superficial peels are appropriate for improvement of skin texture and superficial dyschromias. Medium-depth peels are the peel of choice for the periorbital area due to reliability and predictability and minimal amount of side effects. Deep peels often have dramatic results but accompanied by with longer healing times but are at increased risk for complications. Consistent results are achieved with appropriate patient evaluation and proper peel selection. Having a sound knowledge of chemical wounding and its effects on skin and the post-peel healing process is paramount to avoid complications. Chemical peels can be combined with other adjunctive modalities to improve the quality of skin in the periorbital area.

## References


1. Brody HJ. History of chemical peels. In: Brody HJ, editor. Chemical peeling. St. Louis: Mosby-Year Book; 1992. p. 1–5.
2. Clark E, Scerri L. Superficial and medium-depth chemical peels. Clin Dermatol. 2008;26(2):209–18.
3. Morrow DM. Chemical peeling of eyelids and periorbital area. J Dermatol Surg Oncol. 1992;18(2):102–10.
4. Glavas IP, Purewal BK. Noninvasive techniques in periorbital rejuvenation. Facial Plast Surg. 2007;23(3):162–7.
5. El-Domyati M, Attia S, Saleh FY, Ahmad HM, Uitto JJ. Trichloroacetic acid peeling versus dermabrasion: a histometric, immunohistochemical and ultrastructural comparison. Dermatol Surg. 2004;30(2 Pt 1):179–88.
6. Monheit GD, Chastain MA. Chemical peels. Facial Plast Surg Clin North Am. 2001;9(2):239–55. viii.
7. Brody HJ. Variations and comparisons in medium-depth chemical peeling. J Dermatol Surg Oncol. 1989;15(9):953–63.
8. Monheit GD. Medium-depth peels. Dermatol Clin. 2001;19(3):413–25. vii.
9. Monheit GD. Combination medium-depth peeling of the skin: the Jessner's and TCA peel. Facial Plast Surg. 1996;12(2):117–24.
10. Brody HJ, Hailey CW. Medium-depth peeling of the skin: a variation of superficial chemosurgery. J Dermatol Surg Oncol. 1986;12(12):1268–75.
11. Landau M. Chemical peels. Clin Dermatol. 2008;26(2):200–8.
12. Camacho FM. Medium-depth and deep chemical peels. J Cosmet Dermatol. 2005;4(2):117–28.
13. Herbig K, Trussler AP, Khosla RK, Rohrich RJ. Combination Jessner's solution and trichloroacetic acid chemical peel technique and outcomes. Plast Reconstr Surg. 2009;124(3):955–64.
14. Manaloto RM, Alster TS. Periorbital rejuvenation: a review of dermatologic treatments. Dermatol Surg. 1999;25(1):1–9. Review.
15. Landau M. Combination of chemical peelings with botulinum toxin injections and dermal fillers. J Cosmet Dermatol. 2006;5(2):121–6.
16. Morgenstern KE, Foster JA. Advances in cosmetic oculoplastic surgery. Curr Opin Opthalmol. 2002;13(5):324–30.
17. Kadhim KA, Al-Waiz M. Treatment of periorbital wrinkles by repeated medium-depth chemical peels in dark skinned individuals. J Cosmet Dermatol. 2005;4:18–22.
18. Mangat DS, Tansavatdi K, Garlich P. Current chemical peels and other resurfacing techniques. Facial Plast Surg. 2011;27(1):35–49.
19. Brody HJ. Complications of chemical peeling. J Dermatol Surg Oncol. 1989;15(9):1010–9.
20. Vagotis FL, Brundage SR. Histologic study of dermabrasion and chemical peel in an animal model after pretreatment with Retin-A. Aesthetic Plast Surg. 1995;19:243–6.
21. Hevia O, Nemeth AJ, Taylor JR. Tretinoin accelerates healing after trichloroacetic acid chemical peel. Arch Dermatol. 1991;127(5):678–82.
22. McCollough EG, Hillman Jr RA. Chemical face peel. Otolaryngol Clin North Am. 1980;13(2):353–65.
23. Brody HJ. Complications of chemical resurfacing. Dermatol Clin. 2001;19(3):427–38. vii–viii. Review.
24. Wojno T, Tenzel R. Lower eyelid ectropion following chemical face peeling. Opthalmic Surg. 1984;15(7):596–7.
25. Collins PS. The chemical peel. Clin Dermatol. 1987;5(4):57–74. Review.
26. Dodenhoff TG. Transconjunctival blepharoplasty: further applications and adjuncts. Aesthetic Plast Surg. 1995;19(6):511–7.
27. McKinney P, Zukowski ML, Mossie R. The fourth option: a novel approach to lower-lid blepharoplasty. Aesthetic Plast Surg. 1991;15:293–6.
28. Gatti JE. Eyelid phenol peel: an important adjunct to blepharoplasty. Ann Plast Surg. 2008;60(1):14–8. discussion 19–20.
29. Litton C, Szachowicz 2nd EH, Trinidad GP. Present day status of the chemical peel. Aesthetic Plast Surg. 1986;10(1):1–7.
30. Carruthers A, Carruthers J. Cosmetic uses of botulinum A exotoxin. Adv Dermatol. 1997;12:325–47. discussion 348. Review.

# Periorbital Lasers

4

Jason N. Pozner and Megan C. Jack

## Introduction and History

Rejuvenation of the periorbital area has evolved from purely excisional therapy that often changed one's eyelid shape and led to an aged, hollowed out appearance to a variety of techniques that preserved fullness and a more natural appearance. We have learned to avoid removal of too much fat from the upper and lower eyelids so as to maintain a full, youthful orbit. More controversial is avoiding incising through the lower eyelid orbicularis muscle if possible. The fact that there are so many techniques available for periorbital rejuvenation really means that there is no perfect technique for all people. The introduction of new devices and evolution of others have given physicians a plethora of less invasive options. The introduction of fillers such as hyaluronic acid used in the periorbital area allowed us instant gratification and even more options. The question is when to choose various techniques and which patients are suitable for each device. This chapter will review the use of lasers and other devices for periorbital rejuvenation and their use in combination with surgical procedures.

Electronic supplementary material The online version of this chapter (doi:10.1007/978-1-4614-8388-5_4) contains supplementary material, which is available to authorized users.

J.N. Pozner, M.D. (✉) • M.C. Jack, M.D.
Sanctuary Medical Aesthetic Center, 4800 N. Federal Highway, C101, Boca Raton, FL 33431, USA
e-mail: drpozner@sanctuarymedical.com

Nonsurgical skin rejuvenation is usually thought of in two broad categories—those that remove layers of skin and those that tighten skin without removing any layers. Removing layers of skin can be accomplished with dermabrasion, chemical peels, or lasers. Dermabrasion mechanically removes the top few layers of skin in a relatively controlled fashion, typically using a rotating burr; it is not generally considered an option for periorbital resurfacing due to the thin skin and mobility of the tissues [1]. Chemical peels remove the epidermis and/or a portion of the dermis using a chemical solution applied to the skin and have been used for decades for periocular rejuvenation. Chemical peels come in many combinations and strengths resulting in a range of options for superficial to deep treatments [2, 3]. Laser treatment of the periorbital area began in the mid-1990s with full-field (100 % treatment area; Fig. 4.1) carbon dioxide laser resurfacing and became very popular. These devices allowed for more precise injury, potential for less penetration compared to peels, and provided that added benefit of collagen shrinkage and dermal remodeling resulting in improvement in irregularities and more youthful skin [4, 5]. Erbium lasers and yttrium–scandium–gallium–garnet (YSGG) lasers in full-field mode were introduced and are still in use today. The introduction of fractional lasers allowed us to treat a portion or "fraction" of the skin at any time (Fig. 4.2). The initial devices were *non-ablative* in which a core of desiccated skin was created and caused the body to create new collagen and

S.A. Myint (ed.), *Nonsurgical Peri-orbital Rejuvenation*, DOI 10.1007/978-1-4614-8388-5_4,

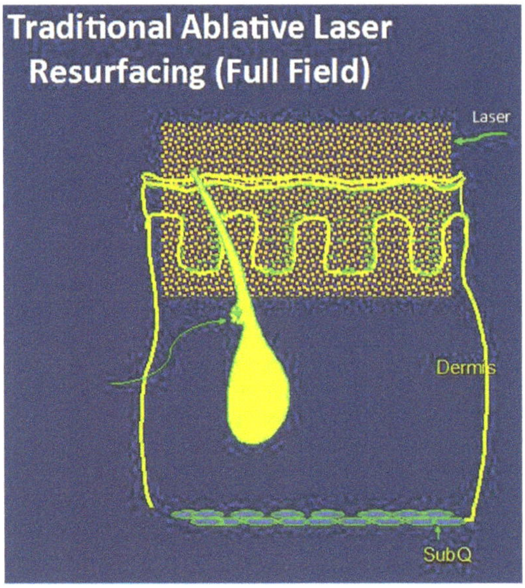


**Fig. 4.1** This graphic illustrates full-field ablative laser resurfacing where 100 % of the surface area is treated in a single session. The stippled area represents the treated area of the skin. Several passes may be required to achieve the desired treatment depth

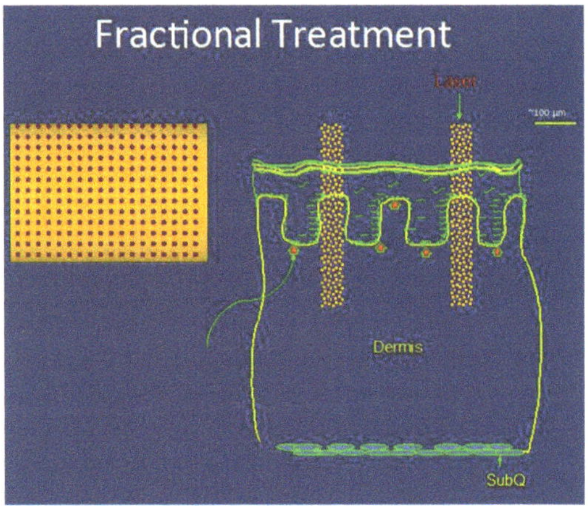


**Fig. 4.2** This graphic illustrates *non-ablative* fractional resurfacing, in which a column of desiccated tissue is created; shown from above (*left*) and side view (*right*). The *red circles* on the *left image* and *stippled area* on the *right image* represent corresponding areas of treated skin. The density of treatment areas can be altered by adjusting the laser settings; typically a single pass is performed at each treatment session

elastic fibers (Fig. 4.2). *Ablative* fractional lasers were later introduced with different wavelengths that removed a core of tissue with some adjacent

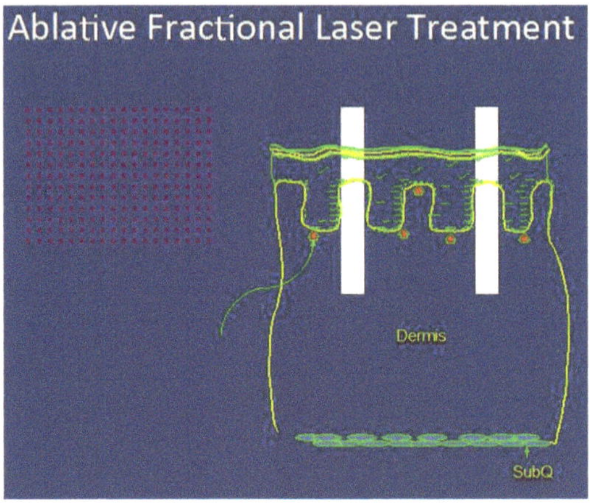


**Fig. 4.3** A graphic illustration of *ablative* fractional resurfacing, where a column of skin (*red dots* on *left*; *white columns* on *right*) is actually removed. Shown from above (*left*) and side view (*right*).

thermal damage (Fig. 4.3). Devices that tighten without removing any layers of skin were introduced in the early 2000s and have been refined since that time. Tightening-only devices include lasers, pulsed light, radiofrequency, ultrasound, and devices that combine two or more of these technologies. Early in their history, most of these devices were not used in the periorbital area as the applicators and hand pieces were too large. Recently, however, some devices were introduced with specific periorbital applications and these will be discussed. As this technology continues to evolve and improve, we continue to expand our capability to successfully treat periorbital aging through nonsurgical means.

## Anatomy

The eyelid skin is the thinnest in the body with epidermal thickness approximating 50 microns (μ) and dermal thickness about 300 μ. The skin thickens as it nears the brow in the upper lid and near the cheek in the lower lid. The subcutaneous layer of fat normally present deep to the skin is sparse in preseptal and periorbital skin and absent beneath the pretarsal skin. However, Asian and Mediterranean patients may have thicker skin and device settings may need to be adjusted accordingly [6].

The sensory innervation to the upper eyelid originates from branches of the ophthalmic division of the trigeminal nerve ($V_1$) which travels through the superior orbital fissure [7]. This nerve provides three branches including the lacrimal nerve to the lateral upper lid and frontal nerve giving off the supraorbital and supratrochlear nerves supplying the medial eyelid. The third nasociliary branch supplies non-eyelid periorbital structures. The lower eyelid sensory innervation is supplied by the maxillary division of the trigeminal nerve ($V_2$) by its terminal branch, the infraorbital nerve via the infraorbital foramen [7].

## Indications

For periorbital resurfacing, lasers are used to remove fine lines and wrinkles through epidermal and dermal ablation and to tighten skin via the body's natural wound-healing response. In comparison to traditional blepharoplasty techniques, laser rejuvenation treats the actual skin elasticity and the eyelid architecture is not affected. Transconjunctival lower lid blepharoplasty and skin pinch blepharoplasty may be performed in combination with laser resurfacing/tightening and will be discussed later. Contraindications may include active infection, history of keloids, and previous deep chemical peel.

## Anesthesia

Periocular laser and device procedures may be performed under general anesthesia, intravenous sedation, local anesthesia, topical anesthesia, forced cold air, or nothing depending upon device and setting used. In general, the more aggressive ablation and tightening devices will require a higher level of anesthesia. Often, isolated periorbital laser resurfacing can be performed utilizing regional blocks with local anesthetic agents. Blocking the supra- and infraorbital nerves based on physical examination and basic anatomic principles will typically provide the patient with adequate comfort both intraoperatively and for a few hours postoperatively [8]. It is helpful in situations such as this to also provide conjunctival anesthesia using ocular drops (e.g., tetracaine hydrochloride ophthalmic solution USP 0.5 %, Bausch & Lomb, Inc., Tampa, FL) prior to insertion of lubricated eye shields. However, as with any procedure, the level of required anesthesia will depend upon the overall health of the patient and patient anxiety/pain tolerance.

## Laser Safety

It is imperative that laser safety is maintained for all cases, all patients, and all operating staff. There are excellent published guidelines for laser safety requirements including fire risk, emergency equipment needed, and suction devices for plume [9, 10]. Guidelines include nonflammable surgical prep and drapes, moistening towels/gauze with saline, specially coated instruments that do not reflect laser beams, a Laser Safety Checklist, proper signage around treatment areas, and use only by certified personnel. Operating room staff should be educated on laser safety protocols.

Eye protection for staff is mandatory for lasers and goggle choice is dependent on the wavelength being utilized. Additionally, it is paramount that the patient's eyes be protected from inadvertent laser injury. Most commonly, topical ophthalmic anesthetic is placed within the eye (see section "Anesthesia"), a sterile lubricant is placed on a non-reflective stainless steel intraocular shield, and the shield is carefully placed in each eye beneath the eyelids prior to periocular procedures (Fig. 4.4). The shields are then removed at the conclusion of the case and the eyes are irrigated to remove lubricant. There are numerous suppliers for periocular shields, although we prefer those made by Oculo-Plastik, Inc. (Montreal, QC). Gold shields are sometimes used for light-based heating technologies around the eyes as there is less thermal transmission for these shields. Nonmetal shields (such as plastic) must be avoided for periocular laser procedures. Coverage with specific external (non-intraocular) shields is used when facial but non-periocular procedures are performed.

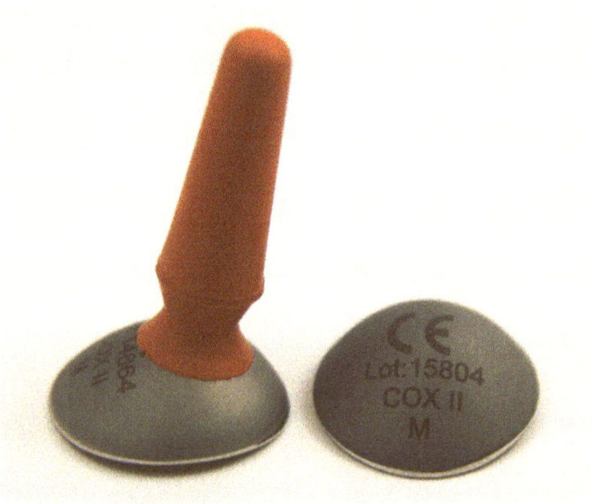


**Fig. 4.4** Stainless steel protective eye shields

## Full-Field Versus Fractional Resurfacing

Full-field resurfacing implies 100 % of the treated area receives ablation and/or ablation plus tissue coagulation (Fig. 4.1). Healing occurs from tissue appendages deep to the injury (e.g., hair follicles). Depth of treatment and amount of ablation and coagulation depend upon laser used and settings. This is compared to fractional treatment in which only a portion or percentage of the area is treated (Figs. 4.2 and 4.3). Full-field resurfacing is used when more dramatic tightening is needed in one treatment, albeit at the cost of longer healing times. By comparison, fractional treatments usually require a series of treatments with shorter healing times. Three lasers are currently in use for full-field resurfacing: carbon dioxide, erbium, and YSGG.

## Carbon Dioxide Full-Field Resurfacing

Carbon dioxide lasers in full-field mode were the first lasers used and popularized for periorbital resurfacing. Their wavelength is 10,600 nanometer (nm) and the chromophore, or tissue target which preferentially absorbs the laser energy, is water. These lasers typically ablate tissue removing about 75 μ and leave behind a layer of residual thermal damage (75–100 μ), but the amount of tissue ablated and amount of thermal damage left behind are ultimately determined by the laser settings used. Initial carbon dioxide systems were used in continuous mode, which generated too much thermal damage and led to unintended sequelae such as scarring. The next generation of carbon dioxide devices was modified to allow shorter amounts of energy to interact with the skin. In the mid-1990s two technologies were in broad use. The Ultrapulse® laser (Lumenis Ltd., Yokneam, Israel) delivered short pulses of light, while the SilkTouch™ and FeatherTouch™ lasers (Lumenis Ltd., Yokneam, Israel) used an opto-mechanical flash scanner to scan a continuous laser beam in a spiral pattern. Both systems allowed short contact time for the laser beam on the skin surface allowing for controlled ablation of tissue and thermal desiccation of a controlled amount of tissue. Current systems use variations of these initial carbon dioxide systems.

## Erbium Full-Field Resurfacing

The erbium/yttrium–aluminum–garnet (YAG) laser (2,940 nm) ablates tissue more efficiently and leaves less residual thermal damage (5–10 μ) than the carbon dioxide laser, as it has an absorption coefficient ten times greater. Because of these attributes, there is essentially a linear relationship between energy density (fluence) delivered and tissue ablated, with 3–4 μ of tissue removed per $J/cm^2$. This means that multiple passes create efficient ablation without additive residual thermal injury. For example, two passes at a setting of 10 $J/cm^2$ are equal to one pass at 20 $J/cm^2$ in terms of tissue ablation depth and residual thermal damage. Superficial and deep resurfacing can be performed using erbium/YAG devices with deeper treatments providing correspondingly increasing results but with longer recovery times.

Variable pulse erbium/YAG systems (Sciton, Inc., Palo Alto, CA) vary the manner in which the laser delivers energy by providing a short ablative erbium pulse followed by longer sub-ablative pulses. The ablative pulse removes tissue while the sub-ablative pulses create controlled thermal damage. These devices can achieve more skin tightening than non-variable pulse width erbium lasers. They allow a varied clinical response with variations in depth of ablation and depth of thermal damage.

## YSGG Full-Field Resurfacing

Similar to the Er/YAG laser at 2,940 nm, the 2,790 nm yttrium–scandium–gallium–garnet or YSGG (Pearl™ Cutera, Inc., Brisbane, CA) has less affinity for water. In full-field mode this device ablates approximately 20–30 μ of tissue and causes residual thermal damage of approximately 20 μ. Multiple passes may be performed to achieve increasing depth of treatment.

## Plasma Resurfacing

Plasma resurfacing systems use radiofrequency energy to convert nitrogen gas into plasma to create tissue ablation and thermal damage. These devices differ from laser resurfacing in that the plasma system creates a coagulated eschar that remains in place as a biological bandage until the skin is reepithelialized. Recovery after a single pass with this device is approximately 7 days. This device was recently reintroduced to the marketplace and may improve mild or moderate facial rhytids, skin color, and skin texture [11–13].

## Fractional Resurfacing

Fractional resurfacing implies that a percentage of the treated area receives laser treatment and a percentage is left untreated. Healing occurs from uninjured tissue lateral and deep to the injured area. As previously described, fractional resurfacing is classified as "non-ablative" in which the device creates a column of desiccated tissue (Fig. 4.2) or "ablative" in which the device *removes* a column of tissue with or without thermal damage (desiccated tissue) lateral or deep to the hole created (Fig. 4.3). Depth of treatment and amount of ablation and coagulation depend upon the laser used and its settings.

## Non-Ablative Fractional Resurfacing

Non-ablative fractional resurfacing was pioneered by Manstein in 2004, with a 1.5 μm prototype laser creating an array of laser micro-exposures called microscopic treatment zones (MTZ) [14]. The original paper discussed treatment of periorbital skin with linear shrinkage of 2.1 % and wrinkle improvement of 18 %. This original research led to development of a number of lasers by varied manufacturers now called non-ablative fractional lasers (Fig. 4.2). The chromophore of these lasers is also water. Wavelengths of these lasers include 1,440, 1,470, 1,540, and 1,550 nm. The devices vary in the width of the thermal zone created and range from 100 to over 400 μ. Overall device power and settings determine the maximum depth of the thermal zone created. The density of treatment is defined by the number of MTZ per $cm^2$. The density and spot size determine the treatment area and may be from under 5–70 % depending upon device, settings, and number of passes performed. When depth is factored in, an idea of the three-dimensional area treated can be ascertained. Epidermal healing occurs very quickly—within 24–72 h—and an inflammatory response is created in the deeper tissue that creates collagen remodeling that lasts weeks to months. Multiple treatments are needed for optimal improvement and usually are performed on a monthly basis, providing skin tightening of 25–62 % or more for most patients [15–17].

## Ablative Fractional Resurfacing

Ablative fractional resurfacing is similar to non-ablative fractional resurfacing in that an array of tissue injury is created by the laser device. The difference being that instead of creating an area of tissue damage, ablative fractional lasers create an

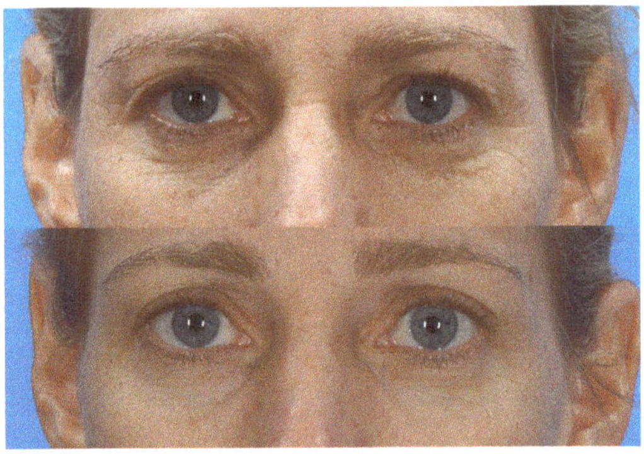

**Fig. 4.5** Patient images showing skin quality before (*top*) and after (*bottom*) fractional variable pulse width erbium laser resurfacing

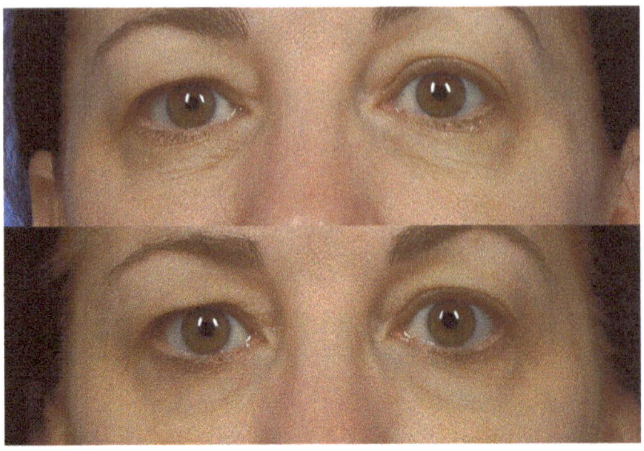

**Fig. 4.6** A 52-year-old patient before (*top*) and 1 year after (*bottom*) a series of four Pellevé® treatments (radiofrequency) to the lower eyelid

area of tissue removal (Fig. 4.3). Three lasers are currently in use for fractional ablative resurfacing—carbon dioxide, erbium, and YSGG. As with full-field resurfacing, these lasers differ in the amount of tissue ablated and amount of residual thermal damage. When comparing periocular fractional treatment of rhytids with carbon dioxide versus erbium, for both modalities wrinkle depth was reduced by 20 % with only one pass [18]. Other authors have reported over 50 % improvement in eyelid rhytids and 42 % reduction in eyelid skin redundancy using slightly more intense laser settings or treatment passes in a single treatment session, and treatments have been found to have long-lasting results [19–21] (Fig. 4.5).

## Radiofrequency

Nonsurgical treatment of the periorbital area with radiofrequency has been shown to improve skin quality and texture [22]. One device on the market, Pellevé® (Ellman International, Inc., Oceanside, NY), is expressly advertised and sold for periorbital rejuvenation (Fig. 4.6). The theory is that the sustained heat from this device causes an inflammatory response and subsequent collagen remodeling [23, 24]. In patients with less photoaging and shallower wrinkles, use of this device in the periorbital region provided 3.5 mm of eyebrow lift, 1.84 mm increase in upper eyelid crease (suggesting tightening), as well as a subjective improvement in periorbital rhytids at 8 weeks [25]. After a series of six treatments, patients were noted to have an average of 50 % improvement which was maintained at 1 year at an average of 30–46 % [26].

## Micro-fractional Ultrasound

Micro-fractional ultrasound is a device that offers both diagnostic and therapeutic ultrasound treatment for skin tightening. This noninvasive device is called Ulthera® and the treatment is Ultherapy® (Ulthera, Inc., Mesa, AZ). The device causes fractional thermal injury to a precisely set depth using ultrasound technology with minimal discomfort and transient erythema [27] (Fig. 4.7). Currently, transducer options are of different depths—4.5 mm, 3 mm, and 1.5 mm. Studies are in progress to evaluate use in the periorbital area. There is a suggestion that the thermal area can be used to either remove fat or perhaps tighten the orbital septum through controlled heat application.

## Laser Treatment Alone for Eyelid Rejuvenation

In patients who suffer from periorbital aging, evidenced by crow's feet, thinning crepey lid skin, and mild to severe rhytids but without a significant amount of excess skin, laser treatment alone can be a very effective treatment modality, offering at least 2.5 years of age reduction [28]. This

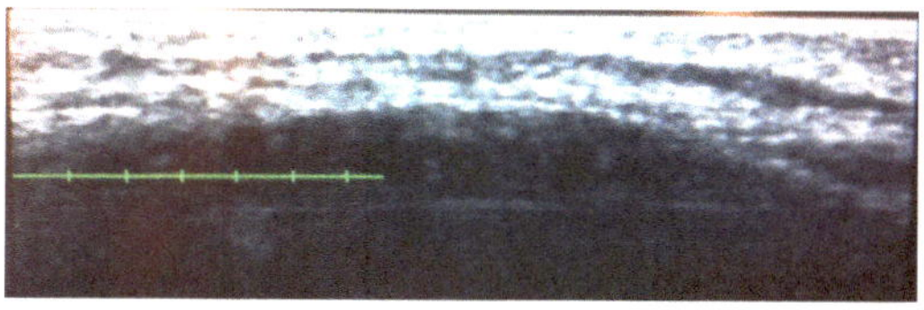

**Fig. 4.7** An example of an ultrasound image of the mid-lower eyelid fat pad utilizing the Ulthera® device during a skin tightening treatment. Note the boney orbital rim (*dark*) with overlying layers of the lid soft tissue (muscle, fat, and skin)

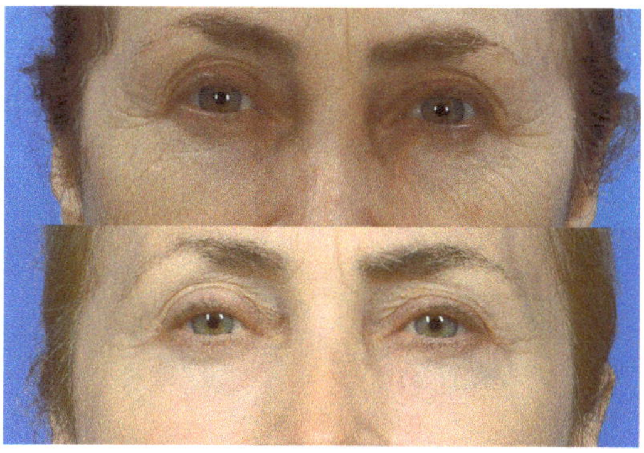

**Fig. 4.8** A 64-year-old patient before (*top*) and 2 years after (*bottom*) full-field resurfacing with variable pulse width erbium laser. Note the improvement in periorbital rhytids as well as skin texture and color

treatment will tighten skin and improve the appearance of rhytids [29].

The question is—what device to use and what settings for that device? As described above most of the early work on periorbital resurfacing was with full-field carbon dioxide devices. The results were very good, but interest in these devices waned after 2000 due to long healing periods and complications including hypopigmentation.

We decide upon device and procedure to be used depending upon pathology and healing time of the patient. For patients with lower eyelid tissue laxity and crepiness, minimal excess skin, skin types I–IV, and enough "downtime" for healing, we prefer full-field resurfacing and have extensive experience with the Sciton, Inc. (Palo Alto, CA), variable pulse width erbium/YAG

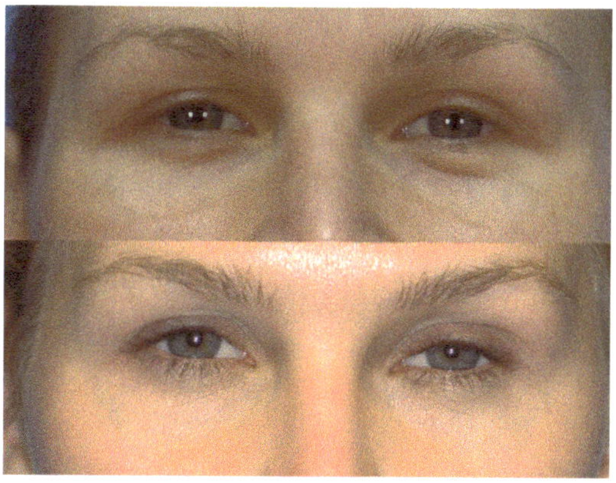

**Fig. 4.9** A 39-year-old patient before (*top*) and 3 years after (*bottom*) laser resurfacing. Note the more youthful appearance to the lower lid skin and tone in this patient

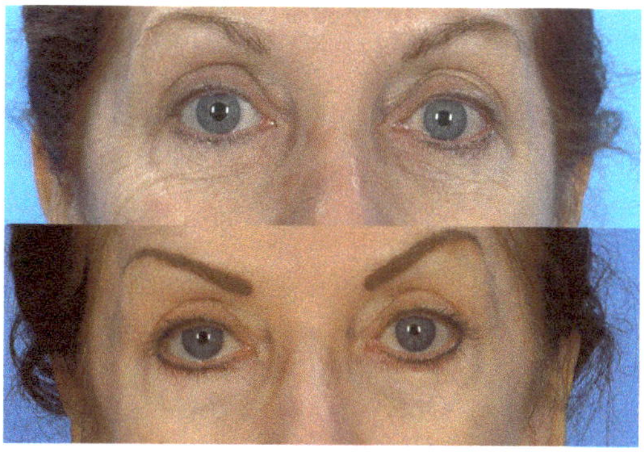

**Fig. 4.10** A 58-year-old patient before (*top*) and 5 years after (*bottom*) full-field resurfacing of the periorbital area with the erbium laser

2,940 nm laser for eyelid resurfacing [30, 31]. Settings vary from patient to patient, but our typical settings are two passes of 80 μ of ablation with 50 μ of coagulation. We treat both upper and lower eyelids with the same settings and treat full upper and lower eyelids to the lash line (Figs. 4.8, 4.9, and 4.10).

For those patients with lower eyelid laxity and crepiness, skin types I–IV, and limited downtime, we prefer an ablative fractional device—either carbon dioxide or variable pulse width erbium.

## Laser Treatment as a Surgical Adjunct

Similar to the integrated treatment of lower eyelids described by Hidalgo using surgery and chemical peels, laser resurfacing is a valuable addition for many patients with periocular aging [32]. Surgical procedures on the eyelid can offer patients an estimated 2-year reduction in apparent age and when combined with the effect of laser resurfacing possibly more [28]. Some authors believe using lasers with blepharoplasty may actually provide better results and shorter downtimes compared with more traditional resurfacing techniques [33, 34].

In most patients with dermatochalasis, skin resection with or without fat removal of the upper eyelids is performed (Fig. 4.11). Adjunctive laser resurfacing with full-field carbon dioxide or variable pulse width laser (erbium) may be performed superiorly and inferiorly to the upper blepharoplasty suture line. Lower eyelid resurfacing is performed as described above. Technically, after upper blepharoplasty is performed, the incision should be closed with a subcuticular suture; we prefer 5-0 polypropylene. After protective laser eye shields are placed, laser resurfacing is performed as above, staying 1–2 mm away from the suture line. Finally, several interrupted nonabsorbable sutures are placed at interval points along the incision to reinforce the closure. It is important to place these sutures after the laser resurfacing so as to avoid burning/melting them and risk problems with the incisional edges separating.

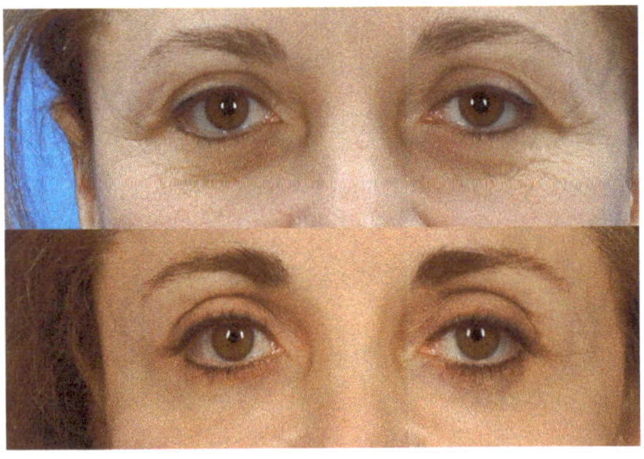

**Fig. 4.11** A 62-year-old patient before (*top*) and 1 year after (*bottom*) variable pulse width erbium laser resurfacing of lower lids with upper blepharoplasty

For lower eyelid rejuvenation, laser resurfacing can be used as an adjunct to transconjunctival blepharoplasty with fat removal or repositioning (Fig. 4.12); it has been shown to decrease the lower lid wrinkling that can actually *increase* after fat removal alone [35]. In some patients with tissue excess beyond the capabilities of the lasers to tighten the skin, a pinch blepharoplasty is typically performed prior to laser resurfacing (Fig. 4.13). As no skin is undermined with these techniques, laser resurfacing can be performed safely concomitantly with surgery and settings do not vary from those used with periorbital rejuvenation with laser alone [36]. Laser resurfacing is performed to the cut edge and then closure is performed with 6-0

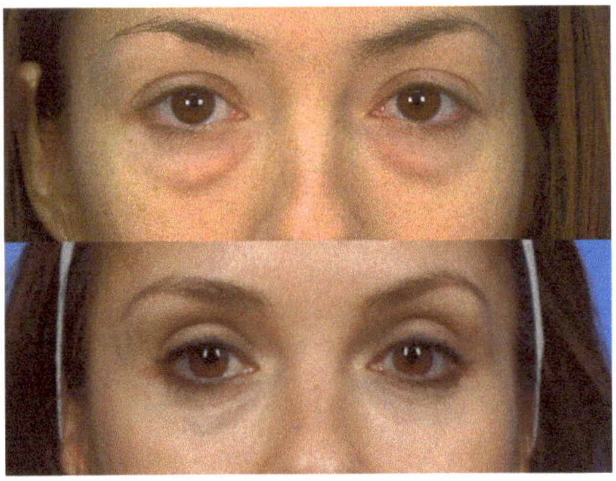

**Fig. 4.12** Before (*top*) and 8-year postoperative image (*bottom*) after lower transconjunctival blepharoplasty with concomitant erbium full-field laser resurfacing to upper and lower eyelids

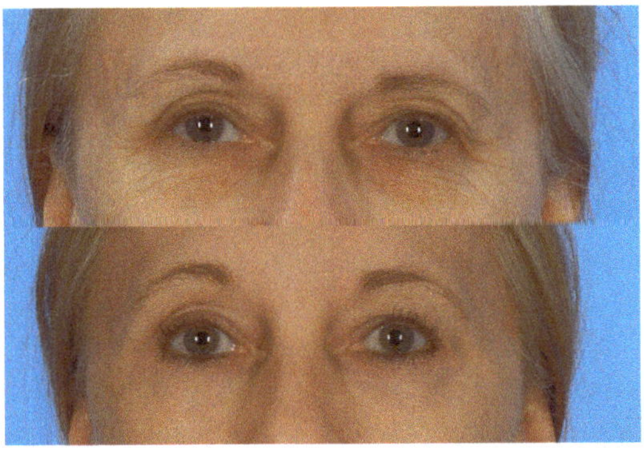

**Fig. 4.13** Before (*top*) and early postoperative patient example (*bottom*). The postoperative view shows 8-month results after pinch blepharoplasty and laser resurfacing with variable pulse width erbium laser

running polypropylene sutures. As described above, closure is performed after laser resurfacing to avoid burning the suture. For those patients with evidence of lower eyelid laxity, a temporary tarsorrhaphy is performed at procedure conclusion to prevent problems with ectropion.

## Patient Assessment

Patients are assessed preoperatively for amount of "downtime" available, expectations, Fitzpatrick skin type, ethnicity, dry eye symptoms or history, degree of skin excess, crepiness, lower eyelid laxity with a snap test, and finances. Based on this assessment and the indications included in the above procedural options, the patient and surgeon choose the most beneficial option. Adequate healing time is necessary for deeper and full-field procedures and needs to be thoroughly discussed with the patient (2 weeks is typical). Laser resurfacing is generally used on patients with Fitzpatrick skin types I–IV, with special attention paid to postoperative management of skin type IV patients to avoid postinflammatory hyperpigmentation. We generally do not perform periocular resurfacing on patients with skin types V and VI. As with any eyelid procedures, care must be taken in patients with history of dry eye. We generally do not perform Schirmer's testing prior to laser resurfacing as it is our impression that the degree of lower lid retraction is minimal to none after laser resurfacing. However, lower lid laxity is assessed with a snap test prior to treatment and patients with poor laxity receive a temporary tarsorrhaphy after resurfacing.

## Step-by-Step: Laser Resurfacing

1. Preoperative assessment is performed as described above.
2. Laser precautions are taken (see section "Laser Safety"). There are many excellent descriptions of laser safety procedures in various publications. Specifically for periocular laser procedures, internal eye shields are mandatory. We prefer brushed stainless steel shields which delay heat absorption (Fig. 4.4; Oculoplastik; Montreal, QC). Topical anesthetic is placed and then the eye shields are coated with sterile ocular ointment then inserted.
3. Anesthesia—Periocular laser resurfacing may be performed under general, intravenous sedation, or local anesthesia. Topical anesthesia is generally not used on eyelids because of risk of corneal irritation. Cold air anesthesia with the Zimmer chiller (LaserMed, LLC; Irvine, CA) alone may be used for superficial resurfacing. If local anesthesia is used, it must be placed after the eye shields; otherwise the shields are difficult to insert.
4. Procedure—Any surgical blepharoplasty procedures are performed first and closed with a subcuticular 5-0 polypropylene suture. Periocular resurfacing is then performed with appropriate settings to the device used (which may vary even between different device manufacturers at the same wavelength) [37]. Our preference is the Sciton, Inc. (Palo Alto, CA), variable pulse width erbium laser (TRL, tunable resurfacing laser). Although settings will vary, our general preferred settings are two passes at 80 μ of ablation with 50 μ of coagulation [38]. Settings may be adjusted higher or lower depending upon the patient's degree of wrinkling and skin thickness. We treat both upper and lower eyelids with the same settings and treat full upper eyelids from brow to lash line and lower eyelids from the lash line to the lid-cheek junction. Lower settings are used to "feather" the lower lid to the cheek. If full face resurfacing is performed, periocular feathering is not needed.
5. Eye shields are removed and lubricant is irrigated out using sterile saline.
6. Suturing is performed of open wounds if lower eyelid pinch is performed or upper eyelid interrupted polypropylene sutures (a few generally placed in the upper eyelid as patients cleaning their skin occasionally pull out their subcuticular suture).
7. Temporary tarsorrhaphy is performed laterally if indicated [39].
8. Occlusive agent such as petrolatum, Aquaphor Healing Ointment (Beiersdorf, Inc., Wilton,

CT), or EltaMD® Laser Post Procedure Balm (Swiss American Products, Carrollton, TX).

## Postoperative Care

There are published descriptions of post-laser care protocols, but here we describe our protocol [40, 41]. Patients are instructed to gently cleanse the treated area three to four times per day with a mixture of 10–12 oz of water and small amounts of Cetaphil® (Galderma Laboratories; Ft Worth, TX) and peroxide. They are seen frequently to assess healing, starting post-procedural day one. Healing times vary with depth of laser resurfacing, being longer for deeper resurfacing procedures. Occlusive agents as mentioned above are applied after cleansing and throughout the day as needed until epithelialization is complete—generally 5–7 days but vary with laser depth of treatment [42]. After reepithelialization, patients are then transitioned to water and Cetaphil® washes and a less occlusive moisturizer, such as EltaMD®. In addition, patients are counseled on the importance of sun protection and are started on a zinc- and titanium-based sunscreen. Eventually, patients are started on one of the many skin care lines available. The typical course of healing for a patient after full-field erbium laser resurfacing can be seen in Fig. 4.14.

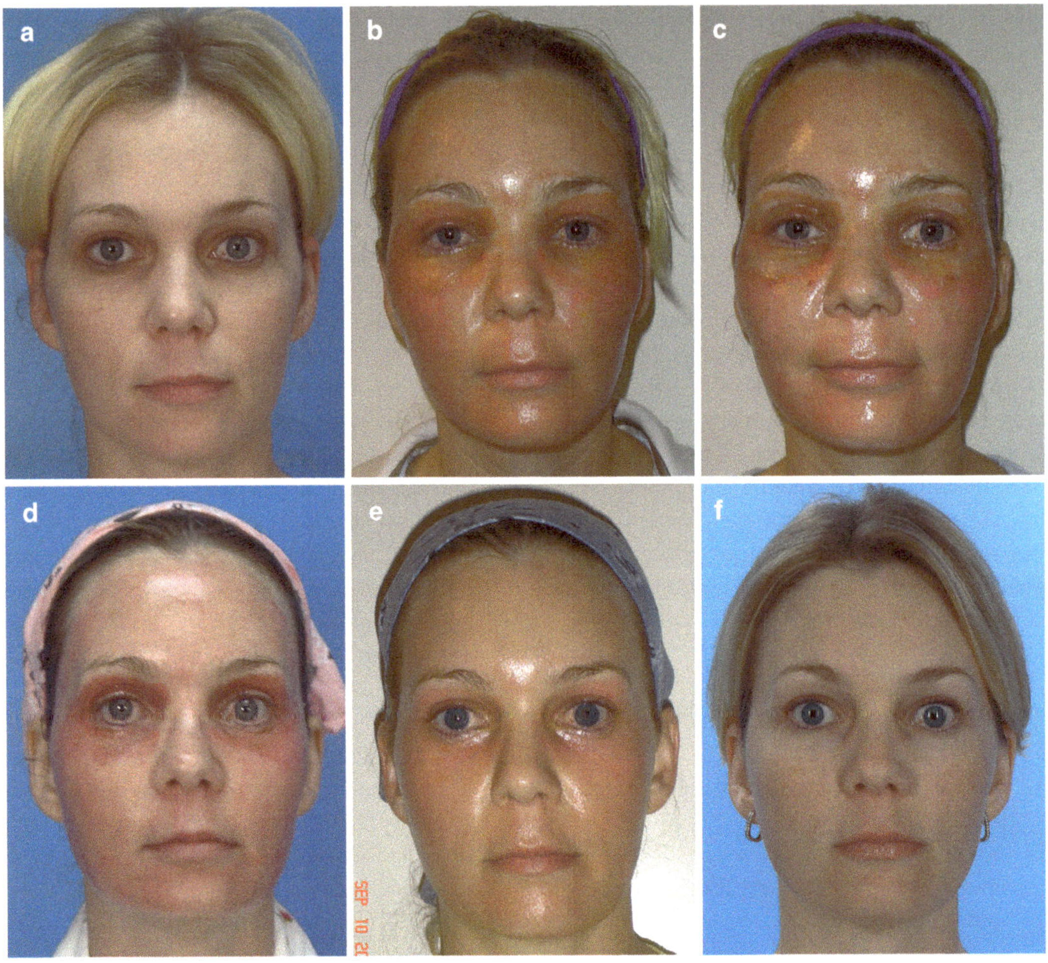


**Fig. 4.14** This series of images shows the typical course of patient healing following full-field variable pulse width erbium laser resurfacing. (**a**) Preoperative; (**b**) 2 days post-laser; (**c**) 3 days post-laser; (**d**) 4 days post-laser; (**e**) 8 days post-laser; (**f**) 6 months post-laser

## Complications

Potential complications associated with laser resurfacing of the eyelids do not differ significantly from those of laser resurfacing in general. Many potential complications may be avoided by a thorough preoperative assessment and appropriate patient selection [43]. The more common laser resurfacing complications include hypo- and hyperpigmentation (either temporary or permanent), prolonged erythema, bacterial/viral/fungal infections, delayed healing, eye injury, and scarring. Viral infection from herpes simplex is a well-known complication, even in patients with no previous history of cold sores. Patients should be provided with appropriate oral antiviral medications before the procedure, and these should be continued for approximately 7–10 days post-procedurally. Rare complications have been described and may include elimination of elastic fibers and resultant violaceous papules [44]. As discussed above in laser safety, general laser risks include fire hazards and protective precautions should be taken to protect all those in the vicinity of laser treatment areas [45].

Synechiae are areas of skin (usually lower lid) that heal together after laser resurfacing (Fig. 4.15). Treatment is to pull these areas apart during the healing period. If allowed to heal, a line may be created with the risk of cyst formation from epidermal occlusion.

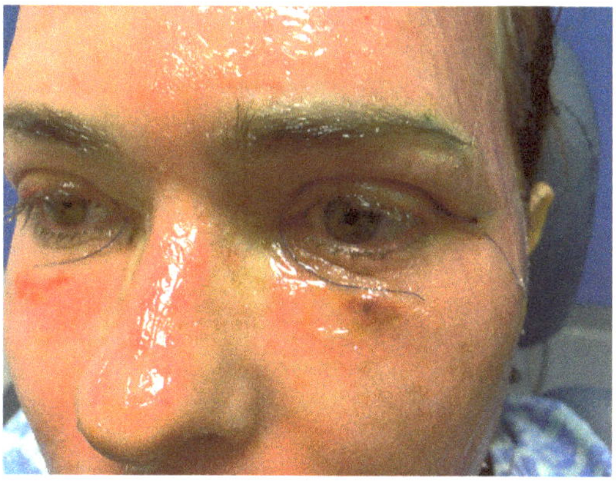

**Fig. 4.15** Example of a potential complication of periorbital laser resurfacing—synechiae—following variable pulse width erbium laser resurfacing

Pigmentation sequelae are more common in patients with darker skin types or tanned skin. Although many providers often avoid laser procedures in patients with Fitzpatrick V–VI class skin, certain precautions can be taken such that some devices can be used [46]. Milia are benign, keratin-filled cysts that often occur as a result of ablative laser resurfacing and can be seen on the eyelids. Although these are not true complications, they can be distressing to patients so should be discussed. These can easily be extracted using a small gauge hypodermic needle in the office should they occur.

Of specific concern with use of laser resurfacing in eyelid rejuvenation, however, are risks such as ectropion and lid malposition, dry eye, retinal injury from the laser itself, and corneal injury from use of the ocular protective shields. Laser treatment of periorbital rhytids is not an exception to the well-described risks associated with periorbital rejuvenation in general [47]. Overly aggressive treatment in sensitive areas such as the periocular region or persistent post-treatment infection may result in permanent scarring and exposure keratopathy [48, 49]. Patients need to be evaluated with respect to brow position, lid laxity, dry eye symptoms, visual disturbance, lid asymmetry, scleral show, and a negative vector. Positive findings need to be addressed preoperatively and a discussion must ensue regarding how such a positive finding may impact results and risks. It is important to discuss asymmetry with the patient as such findings may be more noticeable to the patient post-procedurally and attempts at intraoperative correction can be discussed. Precautions should be taken to protect the patient from undue risk and to avoid complications for these elective procedures. For example, as discussed in patients with lower lid laxity, we place a temporary tarsorrhaphy suture after performing the laser portion of any periocular rejuvenation procedure. If there is any question, refer the patient for ophthalmologic evaluation for a preoperative recommendation.

## Conclusion

Periorbital rejuvenation has advanced by leaps and bounds since its inception and continues to improve as new technologies become available. Despite excellent surgical technique and results, for some patients surgery alone does not achieve their aesthetic goal and adjunct procedures are required. A number of authors have described the benefit of two-pronged approach (surgical and nonsurgical) in such patients [32, 50–52]. However, the plethora of treatment options may cause some confusion for practitioners who do not perform these procedures on a regular basis. It is important to learn about the available treatment options and familiarize yourself with the indications, risks, and technical aspects of the procedure prior to attempting them on your own [2, 53–57]. Surgery for periorbital rejuvenation will always be important; however, laser resurfacing procedures are an extremely useful tool to have for use either alone or in conjunction with surgery.

## References


1. Baker TM. Dermabrasion: as a complement to aesthetic surgery. Clin Plast Surg. 1998;25(1):81–8.
2. Deprez P. Textbook of chemical peels: superficial, medium, and deep peels in cosmetic practice. Oxfordshire: Taylor & Francis; 2007.
3. Baker TJ, editor. Skin resurfacing. Clin Plast Surg. 1998;25(1):1–53
4. Fulton Jr JE, Barnes T. Collagen shrinkage (selective dermaplasty) with the high-energy pulsed carbon dioxide laser. Dermatol Surg. 1998;24(1):37–41.
5. Felder DS. $CO_2$ laser skin resurfacing in oculoplastic surgery. Curr Opin Opthalmol. 1996;7(5):32–7.
6. Kang DH, Choi JH, Koo SH, Park SH. Laser blepharoplasty in Asians. Ann Plast Surg. 2002;48(3): 246–51.
7. Gladstone GJ, Black EH, Rose Jr JG, Sierra CA, Myint S, Brazzo BG, et al. Oculoplastic surgery atlas: eyelid disorders. New York: Springer; 2002.
8. Ismail AR, Anthony T, Mordant DJ, MacLean H. Regional nerve clock of the upper eyelid in oculoplastic surgery. Eur J Ophthalmol. 2006;16(4):509–13.
9. American Society for Laser Medicine and Surgery: Wausau, WI. http://www.aslms.org/professional/.
10. American National Standard for Safe Use of Lasers, 2011; ANSI Z136.3. Laser Institute of America. http://www.lia.org/store/ANSI%20Z136%20Standards and www.lasersafety.org/uploads/pdf/Z136_3_s.pdf
11. Bentkover SH. Plasma skin resurfacing: personal experience and long-term results. Facial Plast Surg Clin North Am. 2012;20(2):145–62.
12. Weber SM, Downs BW, Ferraz MB, Wang TD, Cook TA. Facial resurfacing with coblation technology. Medscape J Med. 2007;10(7):155.
13. Kilmer S, Semchyshyn N, Shah G, Fitzpatrick R. A pilot study on the use of a plasma skin regeneration device (Portrait PSR3) in full facial rejuvenation procedures. Lasers Med Sci. 2007;22(2):101–9.
14. Manstein D, Herron GS, Sink RK, Tanner H, Anderson RR. Fractional photothermolysis: a new concept for cutaneous remodeling using microscopic patterns of thermal injury. Lasers Surg Med. 2004; 34(5):426–38.
15. Tierney PE, Hanke CW, Watkins L. Treatment of lower eyelid rhytids and laxity with ablative fractionated carbon-dioxide laser resurfacing: Case series and review of the literature. J Am Acad Dermatol. 2011;64(4):730–40.
16. Sukal SA, Chapas AM, Bernstein LJ, Hale EK, Kim KH, Geronemus RG. Eyelid tightening and improved eyelid aperture through nonablative fractional resurfacing. Dermatol Surg. 2008;34(11):1454–8.
17. Foster KW, Kouba DJ, Fincher EE, Glicksman ZS, Hayes J, Valerie F, et al. Early improvement in rhytids and skin laxity following treatment with a combination fractional laser emitting two wavelengths sequentially. J Drugs Dermatol. 2008;7(2):108–11.
18. Karsai S, Czarnecka A, Jünger M, Raulin C. Ablative fractional lasers (CO(2) and Er:YAG): a randomized controlled double-blind split-face trial of the treatment of peri-orbital rhytids. Lasers Surg Med. 2010; 42(2):160–7.
19. Kotlus BS. Dual-depth fractional carbon dioxide laser resurfacing for periocular rhytidosis. Dermatol Surg. 2010;36(5):623–8.
20. Mezzana P, Scarinci F, Costantino A, Marabottini N, Valeriani M. Lower eyelid ablative fractional resurfacing: a new technique to treat skin laxity and photoaging. Acta Chir Plast. 2010;52(2–4):35–8.
21. Fitzpatrick RE, Rostan EF, Marchell N. Collagen tightening induced by carbon dioxide laser versus erbium: YAG laser. Lasers Surg Med. 2000;27(5):395–403.
22. Ruiz-Esparza J. Noninvasive lower eyelid blepharoplasty: a new technique using nonablative radiofrequency on periorbital skin. Dermatol Surg. 2004;30 (2 pt 1):125–9.
23. Goldstein SM. Ocular surface temperature changes associated with Pellevé radiofrequency treatment. American Society of Ophthalmic Plastic and Reconstructive Surgery Annual Fall Scientific Symposium Presentation, Oct 2011. http://www.pelleve.com/clinical-publications.html
24. Stampar M. The Pelleve procedure: an effective method for facial wrinkle reduction and skin tightening. Facial Plast Surg Clin North Am. 2011;19(2): 335–45.

25. Javate RM, Cruz RT. Use of an imaging device after nonablative radiofrequency (Pellevé) treatment of periorbital rhytids. American Society of Ophthalmic Plastic and Reconstructive Surgery Annual Fall Scientific Symposium Presentation, Oct 2011. http://www.pelleve.com/clinical-publications.html
26. Taub AF, Tucker RD, Palange A. Facial tightening with an advanced 4-MHz monopolar radiofrequency device. J Drugs Dermatol. 2012;11(11):1288–94.
27. Gliklich RE, White WM, Slayton MH, Barthe PG, Makin IR. Clinical pilot study of intense ultrasound therapy to deep dermal facial skin and subcutaneous tissues. Arch Facial Plast Surg. 2007;9(2):88–95.
28. Swanson E. Objective assessment of change in apparent age after facial rejuvenation. J Plast Reconstr Aesthet Surg. 2011;64(9):1124–31.
29. Alster TS, Bellew SG. Improvement of dermatochalasis and periorbital rhytids with a high-energy pulsed $CO_2$ laser: a retrospective study. Dermatol Surg. 2004;30(4 Pt 1):483–7.
30. Lieb WE, Klink T, Münnich S. $CO_2$ and erbium YAG laser in eyelid surgery. A comparison. Ophthalmologe. 2000;97(12):835–41. German.
31. Millman AL, Mannor GE. Histologic and clinical evaluation of combined eyelid erbium: YAG and $CO_2$ laser resurfacing. Am J Ophthalmol. 1999;127(5): 614–6.
32. Hidalgo DA. An integrated approach to lower blepharoplasty. Plast Reconstr Surg. 2011;127(1):386–95.
33. Kim EM, Bucky LP. Power of the pinch: pinch lower lid blepharoplasty. Ann Plast Surg. 2008;60(5):532–7.
34. Punthakee X, Keller GS, Vose JG, Stout W. New technologies in aesthetic blepharoplasty and brow-lift surgery. Facial Plast Surg. 2010;26(3):260–5.
35. Perkins SW, Batniji RK. Rejuvenation of the lower eyelid complex. Facial Plast Surg. 2005;21(4): 279–85.
36. Carter SR, Seiff SR, Choo PH, Vallabhanath P. Lower eyelid CO(2) laser rejuvenation: a randomized, prospective clinical study. Ophthalmology. 2001;108(3): 437–41.
37. Alster TS. Comparison of two high-energy, pulsed carbon dioxide lasers in the treatment of periorbital rhytids. Dermatol Surg. 1996;22(6):541–5.
38. Harris DM, Fried D, Reinisch L, Bell T, Schachter D, From L, et al. Eyelid resurfacing. Lasers Surg Med. 1999;25(2):107–22.
39. Rosenburg GJ. Temporary tarsorrhaphy suture to prevent or treat scleral show and ectropion secondary to laser resurfacing or laser blepharoplasty. Plast Reconstr Surg. 2000;106(3):726–7.
40. Weinstein C. Postoperative laser care. Clin Plast Surg. 2000;27(2):251–62.
41. Weinstein C, Ramirez OM, Pozner JN. Postoperative care following $CO_2$ laser resurfacing: avoiding pitfalls. Plast Reconstr Surg. 1997;100(7):1855–66.
42. Mannor GE, Phelps RG, Friedman AH, Meltzer M. Eyelid healing after carbon dioxide laser skin resurfacing: histological analysis. Arch Ophthalmol. 1999;117(7):913–6.
43. Weinstein C, Pozner JN, Ramirez OM. Complications of carbon dioxide laser resurfacing and their prevention. Aesthet Surg J. 1997;17(4):216–25.
44. Richert SM, Bridenstine J. Transepidermal elimination of elastic fibers after carbon dioxide laser resurfacing. A report of two cases. Dermatol Surg. 1998;24(2):275–8.
45. Sheinbein DS, Loeb RG. Laser surgery and fire hazards in ear, nose, and throat surgeries. Anesthesiol Clin. 2010;28(3):485–96.
46. Ho SGY, Chan HHL. Laser treatment of ethnic skin. In: Hruza G, Avram M, editors. Lasers and lights. 3rd ed. London: Elsevier Saunders; 2013.
47. Mack WP. Complications in periocular rejuvenation. Facial Plast Surg Clin North Am. 2010;18(3): 435–56.
48. Fife DJ, Fitzpatrick RE, Zachary CB. Complications of fractional $CO_2$ laser resurfacing: four cases. Lasers Surg Med. 2009;41(3):179–84.
49. Mieziak AI, Gottsch JD, Iliff NT. Exposure keratopathy after cosmetic $CO_2$ laser skin resurfacing. Cornea. 2000;19(6):846–8.
50. Trelles MA, Brychta P, Stanex J, Allones I, Alvarez J, Koegler G, et al. Laser techniques associated with facial aesthetic and reparative surgery. Facial Plast Surg. 2005;21(2):83–98.
51. Roberts 3rd TL. The emerging role of laser resurfacing in combination with traditional aesthetic facial plastic surgery. Aesthetic Plast Surg. 1998;22(2): 75–80.
52. Roberts 3rd TL. Laser blepharoplasty and laser resurfacing of the periorbital area. Clin Plast Surg. 1998; 25(1):95–108.
53. Pozner JN, DiBernardo BE, Bass LS. Laser resurfacing. In: Hruza G, Avram M, editors. Lasers and lights. 3rd ed. London: Elsevier Saunders; 2013.
54. Goldberg DJ. Lasers for facial rejuvenation. Am J Clin Dermatol. 2003;4(4):225–34.
55. Papadavid E, Katsambas A. Lasers for facial rejuvenation: a review. Int J Dermatol. 2003;42(6):480–7.
56. Bernstein EF, Andersen D, Zelickson BD. Laser resurfacing for dermal photoaging. Clin Plast Surg. 2000;27(2):221–40.
57. Manaloto RM, Alster TS. Periorbital rejuvenation: a review of dermatologic treatments. Dermatol Surg. 1999;25(1):1–9.

# Radiofrequency/Ultrasound

# 5

Daniel I. Schlessinger, Joel Schlessinger, and Heidi A. Waldorf

## Introduction

Although recent research in cosmetic procedures has allowed for great advances in both surgical and nonsurgical advances in skin rejuvenation, there is a greater demand in the United States for the latter. From 1997 to 2011, the number of surgical procedures nearly doubled from 939,192 to 1,638,524, whereas the number of nonsurgical procedures increased more than tenfold from 740,751 to 7,555,986 [1]. Among members of the American Academy of Facial Plastic and Reconstructive Surgery, the top cosmetic trend in 2011 was the increased use of nonsurgical cosmetic procedures, to essentially delay invasive surgical procedures [2].

There are clear differences between invasive and noninvasive surgical procedures, which lead to some preferential results [3–5] for invasive procedures. Nonetheless, nonsurgical skin rejuvenation procedures allow patients less downtime, quicker procedures, fewer complications, and potentially reduced costs, making them far more desirable to consumers. Furthermore, the ability to undergo these procedures with minimal or no analgesia or anesthetics reduces risk and recovery time further. In this chapter we explore two methods for nonsurgical facial rejuvenation—radiofrequency (RF) and ultrasound. We will focus on the periorbital area, but some discussion includes other facial areas as well.

RF has been a treatment modality for many medical issues, including snoring, liver/lung/kidney tumors, sleep apnea, atrial fibrillation, and back/neck pain [6–12]. It entered the realm of skin rejuvenation in 2002 when the Food and Drug Administration (FDA) approved the first RF device for facial skin tightening, Thermage (Solta, Hayward, CA) [13]. Since then, many different variants of RF devices have been developed and approved by the FDA [14]. A complete list of RF devices currently on the market is presented in Table 5.1. The original protocol for Thermage treatment was for use of about 150 of 1 $cm^2$ pulses at high energies. Thermage subsequently released an updated protocol using multiple pulses (up to 900 on the face) of a larger spot size (3 $cm^2$) at moderate to low energy which provided more efficacy and less pain than the

The original version of this chapter was revised. An erratum to this chapter can be found at DOI 10.1007/978-1-4614-8388-5_8

Electronic supplementary material: The online version of this chapter (doi:10.1007/978-1-4614-8388-5_5) contains supplementary material, which is available to authorized users.

D.I. Schlessinger
Northwestern University School of Medicine, Chicago, IL, USA

J. Schlessinger, MD, FAAD, FAACS
Director, Advanced Skin Research Center, Omaha, NE, USA
e-mail: skindoc@lovelyskin.com

H.A. Waldorf, MD (✉)
Director, Laser & Cosmetic Dermatology, Mount Sinai Medical Center, and Associate Clinical Professor Icahn School of Medicine, New York, NY, USA

Waldorf Dermatology & Laser Associates, PC, Nanuet, NY, USA
e-mail: hwaldorfmd@waldorfderm.com

S.A. Myint (ed.), *Nonsurgical Peri-orbital Rejuvenation*, DOI 10.1007/978-1-4614-8388-5_5,

**Table 5.1** RF devices currently on the market

| Supplier | Product name | Energy source | Energy/power/ frequency | Spot size | Depth of penetration | Cooling method | Ablation |
|---|---|---|---|---|---|---|---|
| BTL Aesthetics | Exilis | Dynamic monopolar RF | 2 W/cm$^2$ | | | Internal cooling | Non-ablative |
| Ellman International | Pellevé | Monopolar RF | 4 MHz | 7.5 mm, 10 mm, 15 mm, 20 mm diameter | | None required | Non-ablative |
| Invasix | Fractora | Bipolar RF | 10–60 mJ/pin | 10×2 pins, 10×6 pins | 500–600 μM | Air cooling optional | Sublative |
| Lumiere Medical and Pollogen Ltd. | Apollo | Monopolar and bipolar RF | 18 W/cm$^2$ | 4×4 mm, 17×17 mm, 87×87 mm | Up to 20 mm | None required | Non-ablative |
| Lutronic | INFINI Microneedle Fractional RF | Bipolar RF | 50 W | 10×10 mm, 5×5 mm | | None required | Sublative |
| | INFINI Superficial Fractional RF | Bipolar RF | 50 W | 20×20 mm, 10×10 mm | | None required | Ablative |
| Solta | Thermage CPT | Monopolar RF | Up to 225 J/cm$^2$ | 2.5×2.5 mm, 15×15 mm, 30×30 mm | | Internal cryogen cooling spray | Non-ablative |
| Syneron and Candela | eMatrix | Diode/bipolar RF | | | | | |
| | eMax/eLaser WRA | Diode/bipolar RF | Up to 50 J/cm$^2$/up to 100 J/cm$^3$ | 12×8 mm | | Internal cooling | Sublative |
| | eMax/eLight SR | Optical energy/bipolar RF | Up to 45 J/cm$^2$/up to 25 J/cm$^3$ | 12×25 mm | | Internal cooling | Sublative |
| | eMax/eLight SRA | Optical energy/bipolar RF | Up to 45 J/cm$^2$/up to 25 J/cm$^3$ | 12×25 mm | | Internal cooling | Sublative |
| | ePrime | Bipolar RF | Up to 84 VRMS | | 1–2 mm | Internal cooling | Sublative |
| Viora | V-touch | Bipolar RF | Up to 25 J | 13.2×13.2 mm, 8×8 mm | 3.9–18.6 mm | Internal cooling | Non-ablative |

original [15–18]. In 2009, Thermage updated its ThermaCool TC device to the Thermage CPT, which utilizes a vibrating handpiece for better pain control and treatment tips with more uniform deep heating allowing treatments without analgesics and with faster seen results [19]. Most recently, Solta launched the "total tip" in May 2013 to provide even more efficient and effective improvement on face and body. These device refinements have led to more patient and physician satisfaction with results.

Ultrasound entered the market in the 1970s with ultrasound-assisted liposuction (UAL) but fell out of favor with various entities, including the American Society for Dermatologic Surgery (ASDS), who issued statements of concern regarding the risk of burns and seromas. While external ultrasound-assisted liposuction was available as early as 2000, this procedure didn't become popular and isn't a widespread technology currently in use.

In 2009, the FDA approved Ultherapy (Ulthera, Inc., Mesa, AZ) as the first external ultrasound device for non-ablative skin tightening of the face and neck areas [20]. This procedure has become very common and is installed in about 1,170 practices worldwide at present [21]. Although use began on the face, the technology is now being used on additional body areas.

This chapter will focus on the Thermage CPT system for radiofrequency and the Ultherapy system for ultrasound. The two other RF technologies with a significant market share, Pellevé (Ellman International, Oceanside, NY) and Exilis (BTL, Boston, MA), will be discussed briefly as well.

## Patient Selection for Noninvasive Tissue Tightening of the Periorbital Forehead and Cheek Areas

Patient selection for these noninvasive tissue tightening of the face and periorbital areas remains the most important indicator of patient outcome. While no hard-and-fast rules are present, generally speaking, patients must be screened for their emotional and physical appropriateness for these procedures. This section will attempt to define the best practices for patient selection.

The best patients for noninvasive procedures such as RF and ultrasound rejuvenation are those who are not ready for surgery medically, emotionally, or financially. In other words, they may have insufficient skin laxity to warrant surgery, have fears of more invasive procedures, or be unable to afford the cost of a large surgery (which often includes operating room and anesthesiology costs in addition to the price of the procedure). Most good candidates are in their thirties to forties and have mild to moderate skin laxity. Older patients who have already had a surgical lifting procedure, have excellent skin quality, or who cannot or will not undergo surgery may also be treated. (Anecdotally the oldest patient one author has treated with radiofrequency tissue tightening was in her early eighties.) Clinically, good candidates for treatment present with periorbital, forehead, jawline, or cheek laxity, marionette lines, pronounced nasolabial folds, and early submental bulging [14].

A major advantage of these therapies is that patients of all skin types can be treated safely even during periods when sun exposure is expected. Although lasers can cause discoloration in patients of Fitzpatrick skin type IV–VI, neither RF nor ultrasound treatments deliver light energy or significant heat to the epidermis and therefore are unlikely to disrupt melanin. Multiple studies have demonstrated the safety of these two treatment modalities for patients with skin of color [5, 15, 22, 23]. The importance of having "color-blind" options can't be understated. Individuals with skin of color are at greater risk of prolonged or even permanent hyper- or hypo-pigmentation after procedures that impact melanocytes. Heat absorption by pigmentation can also lead to secondary blister and scar formation. Because the risk of keloid formation is generally higher in skin of color, surgery is not always a good option.

While treatment is generally safe, there are patients who should not undergo monopolar RF procedures like Thermage. Contraindications for monopolar RF include a pacemaker or any implanted defibrillating device, because the patient must be grounded and becomes part of the circuit. Contraindications for all RF include predisposition to hypertrophic scarring; koebnerization; oral isotretinoin within one year prior; pregnancy; and metallic implants, previously radiation, medical, or cosmetic tattoo (including permanent makeup) in the treatment area. Heating dermal "implants" like tattoo ink can lead to a burn and even scarring. Patients with a history of herpes virus in the area of treatment should be given oral prophylaxis to prevent outbreak [14, 24–26]. It should be noted that RF has been shown to be safe over dermal fillers like hyaluronic acid, calcium hydroxyapatite, or poly-l-lactic acid [27–29]. In the opinion of the authors, care should be taken to avoid edematous, ecchymotic, or non-intact skin because fluence output is based on the device's measurement of skin impedance, so soft tissue augmentation is best performed immediately after, not before, Thermage. However, Dr. Waldorf has treated patients with mild to moderate acne, including cysts, without adverse events (and anecdotally often with improvement). Cysts are treated with intralesional dilute corticosteroids at the time of treatment.

For the Thermage Eyes procedure, metallic ocular eyeshields like those used for laser procedures must be avoided because heated metal can cause ocular injury. Instead plastic ocular eyeshields must be used whenever treatment immediately over the eye itself (rather than over the brow) is planned. No eyeshield should be inserted (and eyes should accordingly not be treated) if a patient has had a recent corneal shield, ocular surgery, or a corneal abrasion, without surgical clearance from that treating physician. Indeed it is generally recommended that patients wait to two or three months to have the eyelids treated with RF after having LASIK surgery [30] unless cleared by their surgeon in advance.

Contraindications for ultrasound include a predisposition to hypertrophic scarring or problems with wound healing. While prior cosmetic or surgical treatments (laser, RF, surgical lifting, or filler injections) are nearly inevitable in the population seeking this form of treatment, as with RF, it is best to wait until any edema or purpura is gone before performing the procedure. Similarly, active skin wounds, severe or cystic acne on the face and/or neck, and infections should be treated in advance. Pregnancy is a contraindication [15, 31, 32]. While any of the above stated issues can be concerning for treatment, many patients are acceptable even with the aforementioned relative contraindications if there is appropriate discussion and consent prior to the procedure. Additionally, the use of fillers such as Restylane, Perlane, or Juvederm prior to the procedure generally isn't a problem if the Ultherapy is being done in other areas. One theoretical risk to the patient is that the fillers may degrade quicker, yet there is no particular harm otherwise.

From a psychological standpoint, a few guidelines have been suggested for patients desiring to undergo tissue tightening. Patients should have realistic expectations about the outcomes, risks, pain levels, and benefits of the procedure. While patients may see some improvement immediately, it should be noted that the most significant results are noticeable 3–6 months after RF or ultrasound treatment. Finally, patients should be completely informed of other options for treatment prior to having surgery [33, 34].

It should be emphasized that the most important contraindication for both of these procedures is that of unrealistic patient expectations. Many patients wish to have a procedure performed that is easy, quick, relatively painless, and has the same or better results than surgery, fillers, or neurotoxins. As part of informed consent, patients must be told clearly that results will not be the same as those achieved by surgery. However, improvements can result with the advantage of gradual natural rejuvenation without downtime, a significant advantage for a large percentage of patients. One of the authors, Dr. Waldorf, specifically avoids calling it a "nonsurgical facelift or eyelift" as a way to stress that results will not be the same degree as those resulting from a facelift or blepharoplasty. She also discusses the treatment as part of a 3-dimensional rejuvenation plan that will also include some combination of neuromodulators, soft tissue augmentation, laser resurfacing, and a good cosmeceutical regimen to maximize results. It is important to show prospective patients not only your best before and after photographs but also more typical examples. If the physician or staff suspects that an individual's expectations cannot be met, it is the physician's responsibility to dissuade the patient and even to refuse to perform the procedure. In the extreme, body dysmorphic syndrome sufferers will rarely, if ever, be pleased by results. Making sure there is sufficient time for both staff and the physician to interact with a new prospective patient is critical for screening. Dissuading someone from a treatment without causing insult can be difficult and can be addressed gently by saying that the procedure is unlikely to fulfill the patients needs.

Pain tolerance and control can also help determine ultimate patient satisfaction. One of the authors, Dr. Schlessinger, gives all Ulthera patients a combination of ibuprofen, Vicodin, and Ativan one-half hour pretreatment. In his experience, Dr. Schlessinger has found injectable anesthetics to be of little or no use because anesthesia is uneven, leading to greater discomfort when painful areas are encountered. He has similar feelings regarding topical anesthetics, since their depth of anesthetization (the superficial aspect of the epidermis and dermis) is not as deep as the ultrasound's depth of penetration (deeper aspect of the dermis and subcutaneous area). On the other hand, the combination of vibration, chilling, and oral pain medications has provided a superior effect with less overall discomfort resulting from injectable or topical anesthetics. Those patients who refuse this combination are dissuaded from undergoing the procedure. In Dr. Waldorf's practice, since the addition of the CPT (comfort pulse technology), Thermage patients no longer require analgesic or amnestic medications, which has resulted in increased patient satisfaction. It was always recommended that topical and injectable anesthetics be avoided with Thermage because of the risk of the hydration and edema altering impedance measurements.

## How Radiofrequency and Ultrasound Technology Play a Role in Eyelid and Facial Rejuvenation

One of many ways to characterize aging is by the loss of collagen, which comprises more than 90 % of the skin's protein. Photodamage is characterized by the accumulation of abnormal elastin (solar elastosis). Occurring at the boundary between the dermis and epidermis, these two processes result in several clinical changes, including skin laxity and the development of fine lines and deeper rhytides [14, 35, 36].

Ablative resurfacing, which includes dermabrasion, Er:YAG and $CO_2$ lasers, and chemical peels, works by causing a controlled zone of damage to the epidermis and dermis and then allowing it to regrow/heal with minimal scarring. Reduction of rhytides and an overall tightening is seen immediately after healing, but additional improvement is noted up to 6 months later. The explanation has been that in addition to the manual resurfacing renewing the epidermis, heat extending to the deeper dermis stimulates new collagen formation. Limitations to ablative resurfacing include a prolonged downtime requiring extensive wound care, the risk of bleeding, infections, unexpected scarring, pigmentary changes, and the need for extended vigilant sun protection [35]. Additionally, Fitzpatrick skin types IV–VI generally cannot be properly treated with laser-assisted ablative resurfacing because of the potential of resulting discoloration and scarring from the light source [5]. These problems led to a goal by physicians and scientists to develop procedures to heat the dermis without affecting the epidermis, including the ones outlined in this chapter.

## Radiofrequency

In ablative resurfacing, the skin's natural resistance (impedance) is a barrier to treatment, as most energy delivered is scattered, reflected, or diffracted, insofar that there is significant energy depletion at the dermis. In contrast, in RF tissue tightening, impedance creates energy by resisting the flow of electrons generated by the device's electric current. Hence, it targets the collagen in the dermis without harming the epidermis. To avoid overheating of the epidermis by the current, a cooling mechanism is usually used at the same time, creating a reverse thermal gradient [14, 19, 20].

Different layers of the soft tissue (dermis, epidermis, fat, fibrous tissue) have different values of impedance [37]. Ohm's Law states that Energy = $I^2 \times R \times T$, where $I$ is current (amperes), $R$ is impedance (ohms), and $T$ is time (seconds). Consequently, more impedance means more energy, heating, and contraction. It also means more potential for wounding [35].

Further, RF energy will follow the path of least resistance. When faced with the choice between adipose tissue and fibrous septae, current will travel through the fibrous septae, which has very similar properties to the dermis. Although fat's resistivity to current is not known, lipids that make up fat are nonconductive. Therefore, current will primarily heat the fibrous septae, which is the reigning explanation for the volumetric heating in the $z$-dimension that is observed with RF devices. As a general rule, fibrous septae heats somewhere between 1.4 and 3 times more than adipose tissue [38]. Additionally, in Thermage CPT, a coupling fluid is used to create a dielectric, which distributes the RF current to create a regional impact rather than a local one [39].

The mechanism of neocollagenesis via RF has been studied in bovine models and seems to be twofold. Analysis by light and electron microscopes demonstrates an initial, immediate collagen denaturation (melting and breaking of its triple-helix) and tissue contraction followed by a lengthier, thermally induced dermal wounding process. The latter process also is thought to stimulate neocollagenesis [18]. It is well documented that neocollagenesis occurs around 65–75 °C [40–44].

RF devices send an electric current between two poles. Some devices, termed monopolar, have one pole on the device and a grounding pole that is placed on the patient's body. Unipolar devices deliver energy in all directions from only one pole, similarly to how a cellular tower sends out a cell signal [14]. Bipolar devices, on the other hand, deliver energy between two poles which are next to one another on the device [24].

Several studies have demonstrated the efficacy of radiofrequency in treating periorbital rhytides and the cheek area. Fitzpatrick et al. treated 86 patients age 35–70 with a single pass of ThermaCool TC in the periorbital area, with energy ranging from 52 to 220 J. Side effects included erythema (36.0 % incidence immediately and 16.7 % within 72 h) and edema (13.9 % immediately and 6.4 % within 72 h). No third-degree burns were observed, and the overall second-degree burn rate was 0.36 %. At 6 months posttreatment, blinded raters determined at least 0.5 mm brow-lifting in 60.5 % of eyebrows and at least a 1-point facial wrinkle scale improvement in 83.2 % of participants [45].

Narins and Narins treated 17 patients age 42–60 with two passes of ThermaCool TC for the full face, with energy ranging from 125 to 144 J/cm$^2$. Side effects included mild erythema which lasted for a few hours. No objective improvement metrics were employed, but gradual improvement was observed in before and after photographs. The low AE incidence rate was attributed to decreasing the energy with any patient discomfort [46].

Abraham et al. treated 35 patients (28 women, 7 men, mean age 51) with a single pass of ThermaCool TC in the periorbital, forehead, and neck areas with energy ranging from 115 to 144 J/cm$^2$. Side effects included immediate mild erythema in most patients, edema in about one-third of patients, discreet, firm, subdermal areas on the neck in 14 % of patients, and transient numbness in 14 % of patients. All side effects subsided within a few weeks of treatment.

Alster and Tanzi treated 50 patients, mean age 53.3, with a single pass of ThermaCool TC with energy ranging from 97 to 144 J/cm$^2$ on the cheek area and 74 to 134 J/cm$^2$ on the neck area. Side effects included immediate mild erythema (average duration of 2.3 h) in most patients, soreness or sensation in 56 % of patients, and erythematous papules in 6 % of patients. All side effects subsided within a few days of treatment. Blinded investigators determined clinical improvement in the cheek area in 28 of 30 patients and improvement in the neck area in 17 of 20 patients [47] (Fig. 5.1).

Bassichis et al. treated 24 patients with a single pass of ThermaCool TC on the upper one-third of the face. These patients were

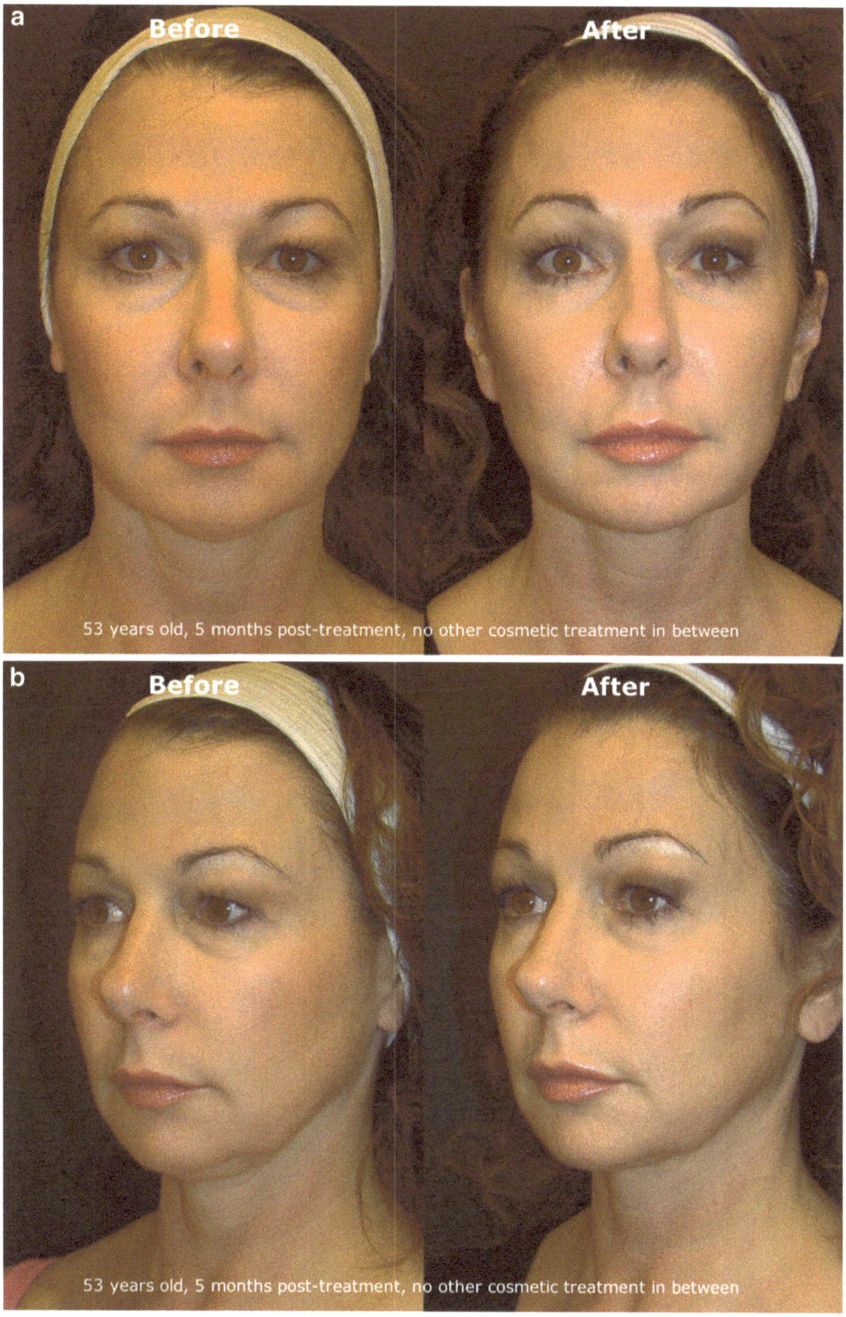


**Fig. 5.1** 53 years old, 5 months posttreatment, no other cosmetic treatment in between ((**a**) Front, (**b**) angled left, (**c**) left side, (**d**) angled right, (**e**) right side)

compared to a control group of 12 subjects. No side effects were noted. Objective brow analysis showed at least 0.5 mm improvement in more than 87.5 % of patients, and posttreatment improvement was statistically significant over the control ($P<0.05$). Patients' subjective self-evaluation and satisfaction levels, however, did not correlate with the objective measurements. Additionally, asymmetry in brow improvement was noted in many patients [48].

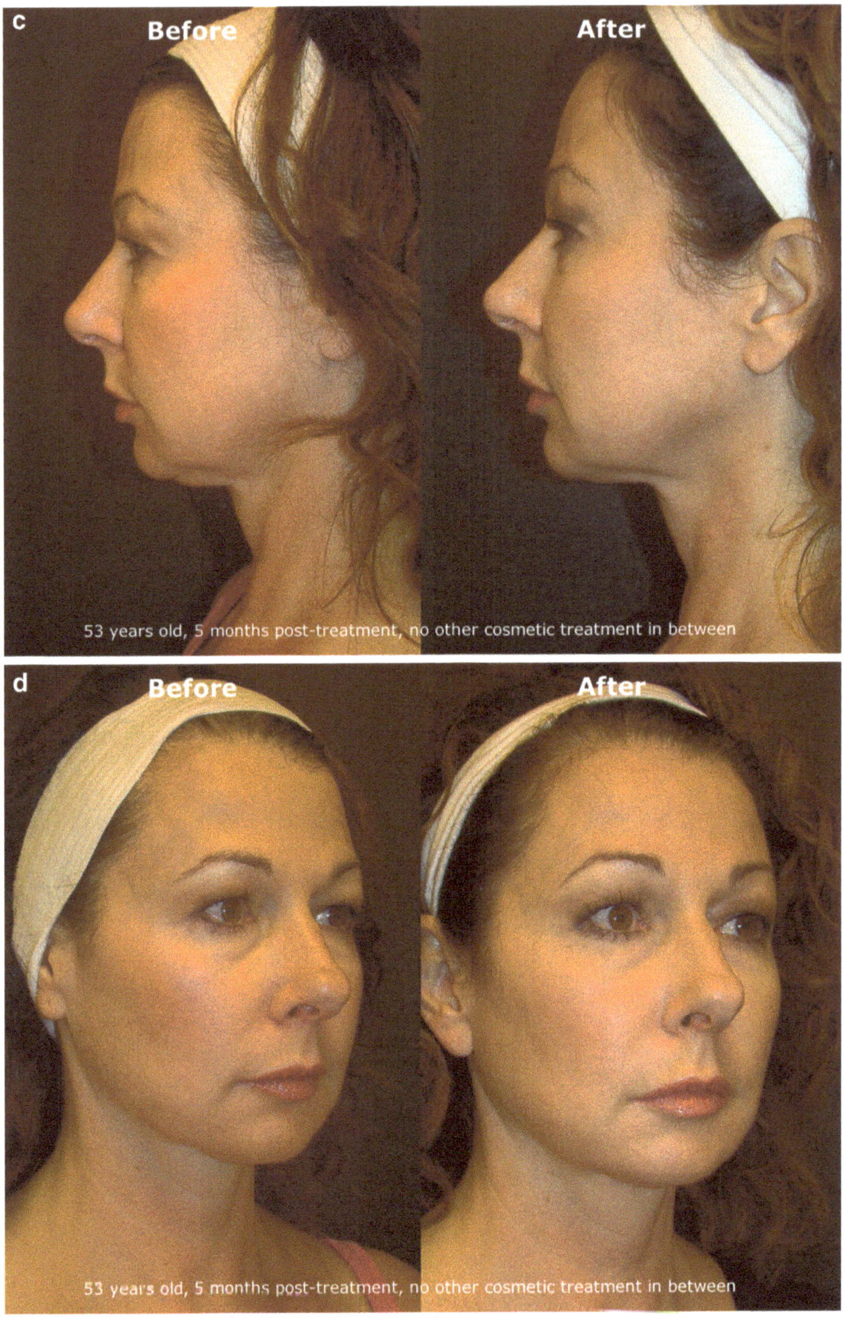


**Fig. 5.1** (continued)

Fritz et al. treated 11 patients with a single treatment and 9 patients with two treatments of ThermaCool TC spaced 1 month apart, on the middle and lower face areas, with energy ranging from 85 to 135 J/cm$^2$. Side effects included mild edema and mild to moderate erythema. All side effects subsided within a few days of treatment. Blinded investigators determined statistically significant better improvements in the treatment group receiving two treatments in the following

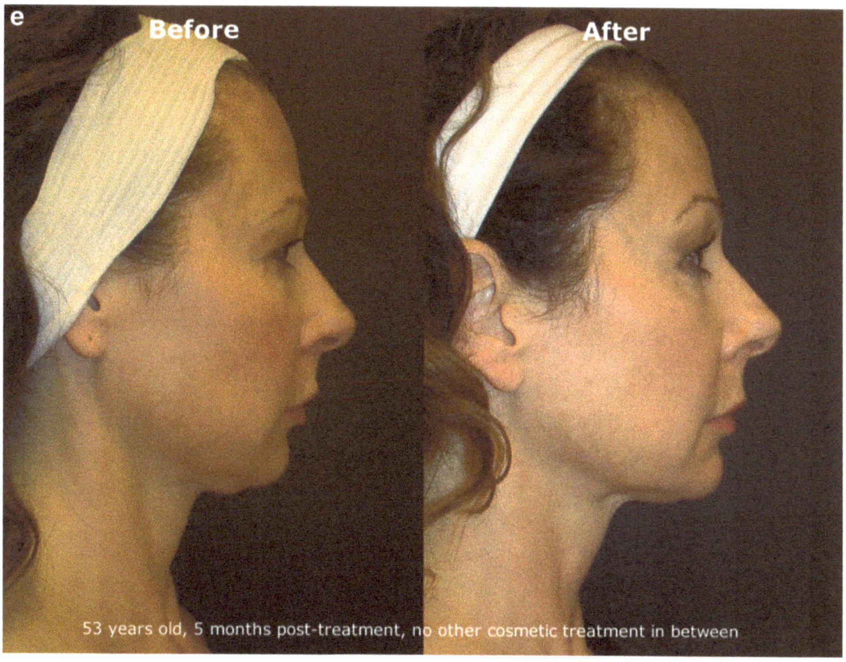


**Fig. 5.1** (continued)

categories: nasolabial folds ($P=0.03$), patient self-assessment ($P=0.04$), and physician photographic assessment at both 1 and 4 months ($P=0.05$). 75 % of subjects indicated they would consider paying for more treatments [49]. With the newest generation of Thermage CPT, post-treatment erythema, edema, and nodularity are no longer expected. With appropriate skin cleansing, liberal use of coupling fluid, and use of multiple passes at medium heats without pulse stacking, blisters and burns should not occur.

## Ultrasound

Ultrasound can propagate energy into the body in such a way that the lower the frequency, the deeper the penetration and vice versa. It is widely accepted as an extremely safe method of fetal imaging. When the same machine is used at a much higher energy, its waves are able to focus to target a very confined region (about 1 $mm^3$). This is the basis for intensive ultrasound (IUS). It has long been known that at these settings, ultrasound can cause coagulative necrosis. It is believed that the intense focus of the ultrasound beam causes vibration of molecules at the target, heating the tissue. Using this knowledge, scientists have begun using ultrasound technology to treat tumors of the liver, breast, and uterus [40, 50, 51].

Other cosmetic applications of ultrasound have been developed harnessing the controllable depth and geometry of IUS. Recently, a high-intensity focused ultrasound (HIFU) device for treatment of subcutaneous adipose tissue (SAT) was developed (Liposonix; Solta, Hayward, CA) and approved by the FDA. In clinical trials, it was proven to be safe and effective for treatment of SAT, reducing waist circumference by 4–5 cm and exhibiting an adverse event (AE) profile similar to sham treatment [52–56]. The same science is the basis for Ultherapy, but Ultherapy is focused deep to the SAT.

In ablative resurfacing, the aim is to create thermal injury zones (TIZs), which then generate new collagen during their repair process. This is a relatively superficial process, aiding the uppermost layers of the skin but not inducing larger structural changes. In contrast, in ultrasound skin tightening, the aim is to create TIZs in the skin's deeper structural layers, inducing greater textural changes. The target of Ultherapy is a layer of the skin called the superficial musculoaponeurotic system (SMAS). Located below the dermis, the SMAS is a fibrous envelope composed of collagen and elastin that communicates muscle movements so that facial expressions are seen in the skin. It is believed that creating TIZs in the SMAS leads to its contraction and shrinkage, as well as collagen denaturation [51].

Several studies have demonstrated the efficaciousness of IUS in contracting the SMAS and rejuvenating the skin. White et al. produced TIZs at specific, controllable depths and sizes in the SMAS of six human cadaveric tissue specimens with IUS. Tissue samples were analyzed with ultrasound before and after treatment and were examined grossly and histologically. Using energy ranging from 0.5 to 8.0 J and combinations of power and exposure times, Ultherapy generated TIZs as deep as 7.8 mm, while preserving the epidermis and surrounding tissues, both superficial and deep to the SMAS [51].

In a separate study, White et al. exposed porcine tissue to IUS using the following probes: 4 MHz, 4.5-mm focal depth; 7 MHz, 4.5-mm focal depth; and 7 MHz, 3.0-mm focal depth. Tissue samples were analyzed with ultrasound before and after treatment and were examined grossly and histologically. It was found that increasing the energy decreased the focus of the TIZs and increasing the frequency decreased the depth of penetration. Using all probes, the epidermis was unaffected [40].

Alam et al. treated 35 patients aged 32–62 with a single pass of IUS for the full face and the neck areas using the following probes: 4 MHz, 4.5-mm focal depth; 7 MHz, 4.5-mm focal depth; and 7 MHz, 3.0-mm focal depth. At 90 days posttreatment, blinded raters judged pre- and posttreatment photographs (which were not categorized as such) for an improvement, worsening, or no change. Additionally, standardized photographs were analyzed for brow improvement using five separate measurement points on each eyebrow, whose brow heights were averaged. Clinically noticeable brow-lifting was seen in 86 % of patients ($P = 0.00001$), and mean average brow change was a lift of 1.7 mm. Additionally, it was determined that the threshold of visible brow change was 0.5 mm change [31].

Lee et al. treated ten patients aged 55–71 with multiple passes of IUS for the face and the neck areas, first with the 4 MHz, 4.5-mm focal depth probe, then with the 7 MHz, 3.0-mm focal depth probe. At 90 days posttreatment, blinded raters judged pre- and posttreatment photographs (which were not categorized as such) for an improvement, worsening, or no change. The patients also were asked to rate their pre- and posttreatment changes. Raters judged improvement in 80 % of participants and 90 % of subjects judged improvement in skin laxity [57] (Fig. 5.2).

## Pretreatment Assessment

### Radiofrequency

Early adopters of Thermage, including one of the authors (Dr. Waldorf), found patients required significant pain management. Topical anesthetic was not recommended because of the risk of changing skin impedance. Narins et al. reported that from October 2003 to February 2004, 70 % of all contour irregularities with ThermaCool TC occurred when nerve blocks and intravenous or tumescent anesthesia were used [58]. It is believed that these pain control treatments, especially intravenous or tumescent anesthesia, decrease efficaciousness of treatment by (1) increasing skin thickness and therefore depth of penetration of RF and (2) providing a potentially dangerous false sense of pain [4, 16, 59]. But some note that extreme discomfort is also a very natural bodily indicator of excessive heating and a sign that treatment should be stopped immediately [4].

After many of the aforementioned discomfort studies were performed, a few modifications were made to the existing Thermage system. The new Thermage CPT system, which sends out alternative vibrations and bursts of cold at unequal intervals through the handpiece, is said to confuse nerves through transcutaneous electrical nerve stimulation (TENS), based on Melzack

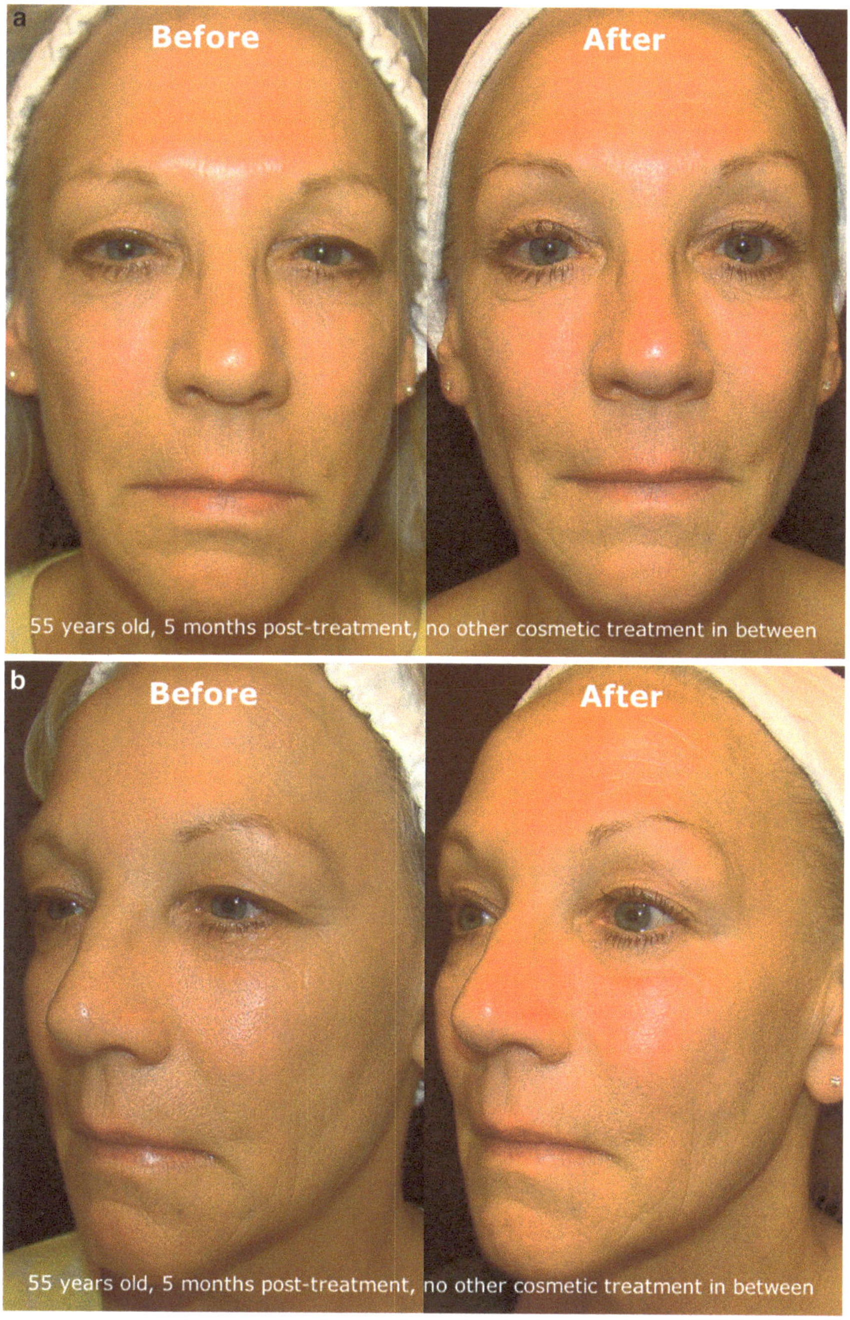


**Fig. 5.2** 55 years old, 5 months posttreatment, no other cosmetic treatment in between ((**a**) Front, (**b**) angled left, (**c**) left side, (**d**) angled right, (**e**) right side)

and Wall's 1965 gate control pain theory. Although there is some evidence that TENS does not actually have any effect on discomfort [60–62], Drs. Waldorf and Schlessinger have found the addition of vibration to treatment areas to be a significant reducer of pain for patients both with the Thermage CPT unit and while using external devices during other procedures. These observations have been supported in the literature [63, 64]. With the Thermage CPT, patients are

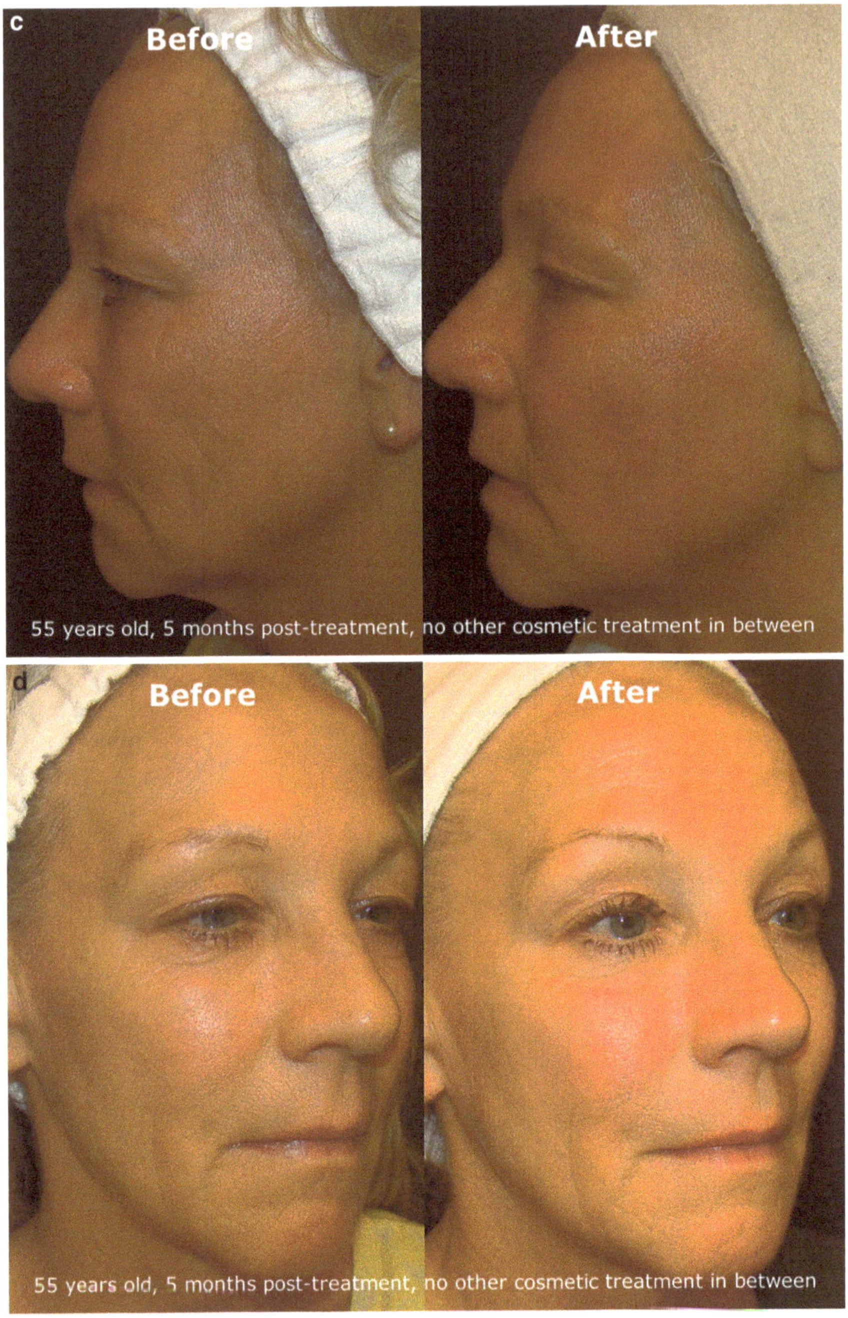


**Fig. 5.2** (continued)

asked to tell the treating staff if pain goes above a level of 2 out of 4. Since upgrading to the CPT system, Dr. Waldorf reports that her patients require no other pain control and routinely comment on the relaxing feeling of the warmth and vibration. If the patient reports pain above a 2 out of 4, if the skin appears red, or if an excessive heat indicator appears, the treating physician or nurse moves to another skin area before returning to that area.

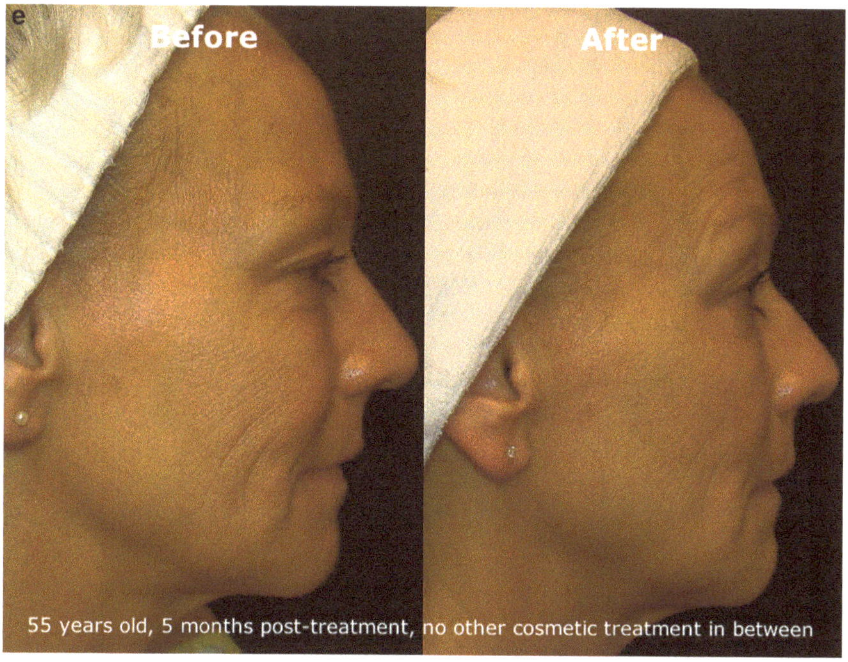


**Fig. 5.2** (continued)

Before treatment, several standardized photographs should be taken. Improvements may be seen better at an angle than face front. Therefore, the authors recommend five standard photographs be taken of each patient: front, 45-degree angle, and 90-degree angle on both right and left. While this can be accomplished with any camera, one system (Canfield; Canfield Scientific, Inc., Fairfield, NJ) features high-resolution camera mounted on a semicircular table that can rotate to take pictures of the face at different angles. It also contains equipment to hold the patient's head in a standard vertical or horizontal pose. While there are many such photographic systems available, this is the system that Dr. Schlessinger and many clinical study investigators utilize to maintain consistency [15, 65, 66]. He also often uses a point-and-shoot camera to take photos, depending on the visibility of the area being treated.

The patient must remove contact lenses and the patient's face must be cleaned of all makeup and creams with a makeup-removing cleanser. Any residue increases the risk of burning by the RF current. It is critical to confirm that all mascara has been removed because coupling fluid can cause it to run and interfere with treatment areas. After makeup is removed, the treatment area should be wiped thoroughly with alcohol (using Q-tips for the eyelids to avoid eye contact). All metal implants and jewelry in or near the area of treatment, including earrings, necklaces, eyebrow rings, and nose rings, must be removed if they can, as they can attract the electric current generated by the radiofrequency device.

One of several standardized grids supplied by the company matching the size of the tip to be used is applied to the skin with additional alcohol, being careful not to get alcohol in the eye. [4]. Current protocols include the 3 $cm^2$ box grids for the face including the forehead and the portion of the upper and lower lids sitting directly on bone and the 0.25 $cm^2$ box grid for the portion of the eyelid resting on the eye itself. The eyelid generally requires 3–4 rows.

If treating the eyelids, protective plastic intraocular shields must be used to prevent current injuring the eyes. It is extremely important that protective metal ocular shields are NOT used because of the risk of heated metal burning the eyes and eyelid. Topical ophthalmic anesthetic drops can be used prior to insertion, but lubricant should be avoided because of the risk of interference with the RF pulses. One of the authors, Dr. Waldorf, recommends inserting an eyeshield only in one eye at a time to avoid patient anxiety. The 0.25 cm tip grid is most easily applied after the intraocular shield is in place to allow the paper to lay flat on the surface to be treated. After treatment of one eyelid, the shield is removed and placed in the contralateral eye and the procedure repeated. Needle-less syringes filled with water are kept available to flush the eyes in case of irritation from alcohol or coupling fluid.

### Ultrasound

Before treatment, the patient's face must be cleaned of all makeup. Male patients should be clean-shaven. All jewelry should be removed, including earrings, necklaces, eyebrow rings, and nose rings. Topical anesthesia, such as EMLA cream, or oral analgesic is usually insufficient for the pain associated with Ultherapy [23, 31, 32, 57, 67] due to the fact that this procedure is deeper in nature. For this reason, it is best to provide oral analgesics such as ibuprofen (800 mg), Vicodin (1–2 in advance), and Ativan (1–2 mg prior) one-half hour prior to treatment.

Clearly, the use of anesthesia will determine the ease of the procedure and patient satisfaction during and after the procedure. For this reason, it is imperative to have a discussion prior to the procedure with the patient.

One important point to note is that if the patient will be given any form of sedation, he or she will have to prearrange transportation for after the procedure. Additionally, any and all consents must be signed prior to the administration of sedatives.

## Procedure in Detail

### Radiofrequency

The device will walk the user through steps including reminding the user of critical steps including placing the grounding pad, maintaining the cryogen, and, for the 0.25 $cm^2$ tip, applying an eyeshield.

Once informed consent and photos are obtained, the skin to be treated is prepared as discussed previously. An adhesive grounding pad is applied and attached to the Thermage device. For eyelid and facial treatment, the pad is generally placed on the mid or lower back. After applying the facial grid, the plastic RF eyeshield and eyelid grid are placed. The underside of plastic eyeshields must be checked before treatment for surface scratches that can cause a corneal abrasion. Coupling fluid is applied and reapplied to keep the skin surface glistening. Once a new tip is placed on the handpiece, impedance of the area to be treated is tested and then treatment level set. The procedure is performed starting at a medium level and pulses applied row by row first in squares and then at the intersection of squares for three or four rows depending on the lid size and avoiding the eyelashes. The level can be raised or lowered based on patient feedback of heat as well as by the treating physician or nurse feeling for heat in the treated skin which should feel warm. The medial or lateral portions of the eyelid can be treated with additional pulses or the entire area treated uniformly depending on the distribution of the patient's laxity. Unless the patient has marked facial asymmetry, half of a tip of 250 0.25 $cm^2$ pulses is used for each eyelid.

After treating the eyelids, therapy moves on to the area of the upper lid immediately under the eyebrow, the forehead, temples, and along the lower orbital rim using the 3 $cm^2$ face or total tip. Again using liberal amounts of coupling fluid, two or three passes are done alternating square and intersection rows followed by additional passes along "vectors" avoiding the eyebrow hair. These vectors are discovered by manually pulling on the patient's skin and then performed as freehanded rows in areas where tightening in a particular directionality can lift the targeted anatomy. These include vertical passes along the lateral forehead, diagonal passes from the glabella upward and laterally, and sweeping passes along the lower orbital rim toward the temple. Pulses should never be stacked to avoid atrophy.

Anecdotally, Dr. Waldorf has found that using a 900 pulse 3 $cm^2$ handpiece for the full face alone, excluding the lid overlying the eye itself, still reduces brow ptosis and lower lid puffiness and tear trough deformity.

Immediately after treatment, the grids are removed with alcohol and sunscreen applied. The disposable grounding pad is removed. The patient can get dressed and return to all normal activities

## Ultrasound

Ultrasound gel is applied to the skin. The probe is then placed gently on the skin to ensure coupling with the epidermis. The device's imaging functionality should be used to ensure the following two conditions are satisfied: the ultrasound energy is acoustically coupled with the skin, and the focal depth of the probe is aiming for the mid-to-deep reticular dermis. Incorrect transducer depth will present as bone in the upper half of the image. If bone is present in the upper half of the image, avoid the area or use a more superficial probe. Poor coupling will present as dark vertical bars on the image, and too much gel will present as a valley at the top of the image. Poor contact with transducer will likely present as darkness on only one side of the image.

For the periorbital area, Dr. Schlessinger starts by marking a border with a white marking pencil at the vertical line of the pupil. For men, the border should be marked about three to four more lines more medial from the pupil to ensure the whole brow is lifted. He then measures ten vertical lines on the Ulthera treatment-planning card with 3 mm in between each parallel line. Another border is made from the lateral canthus to the hairline and five lines are measured above and five lines are measured below from the orbital rim to the hairline. Finally, a curved border is marked along the infraorbital rim and four columns of five lines are measured below (Fig. 5.3).

For the cheek area, it is important to avoid the marginal mandibular nerve, which extends upward from the jawbone to the corners of the mouth. When treating any area around these nerves, leave 1–2 cm of space lateral to the edge of the lips. Dr. Schlessinger marks a curved border perpendicular from the nasolabial folds along the lower edge of the zygoma bone to the upper edge of the ear. Measure columns with the treatment-planning card, starting on the most lateral edge of the cheek. Draw three columns the width of the ruler and measure about 30 lines in each column. Later, when treating with the more superficial probes, it is allowable to treat above the marginal mandibular nerve.

When starting treatment, it is very important to consistently take note of a patient's pain level during the procedure. The energy levels are defaulted to the highest possible treatment—1.20 J for the 4.0 MHz with 4.5 mm focal depth, 1.05 J for the 7.0 MHz with 4.5 mm focal depth, 0.45 J for the 7.0 MHz with 3.0 mm focal depth, and 1.20 J for the 7.0 MHz with 1.5 mm focal depth. The energy level may be adjusted down from these settings. A downward adjustment by one level will reduce discomfort and will not affect the clinical outcome of the procedure.

Treatment begins with a single pulse for the lines in the columns. It is recommended to start with deeper probes (4.0 MHz with 4.5 mm focal depth or 7.0 MHz with 4.5 mm focal depth) for the first pass and move to more superficial probes (7.0 MHz with 3.0 mm focal depth or 10 MHz with 1.5 mm focal depth) for the second pass, as coagulated skin has different thermal properties from untreated skin [68].

After one pass for each side of the face, about 130–150 lines have been delivered. It is then recommended to deliver the second pass with angled lines and with more superficial probes (7.0 MHz with 3.0 mm focal depth or 10 MHz with 1.5 mm focal depth). About 600 lines should be delivered at the end of treatment including the neck and forehead.

## Posttreatment Care

In general, posttreatment care is supportive in nature for Thermage as well as Ultherapy. This is one of the attractive features about noninvasive procedures as opposed to invasive procedures. Erythema following Thermage generally resolves

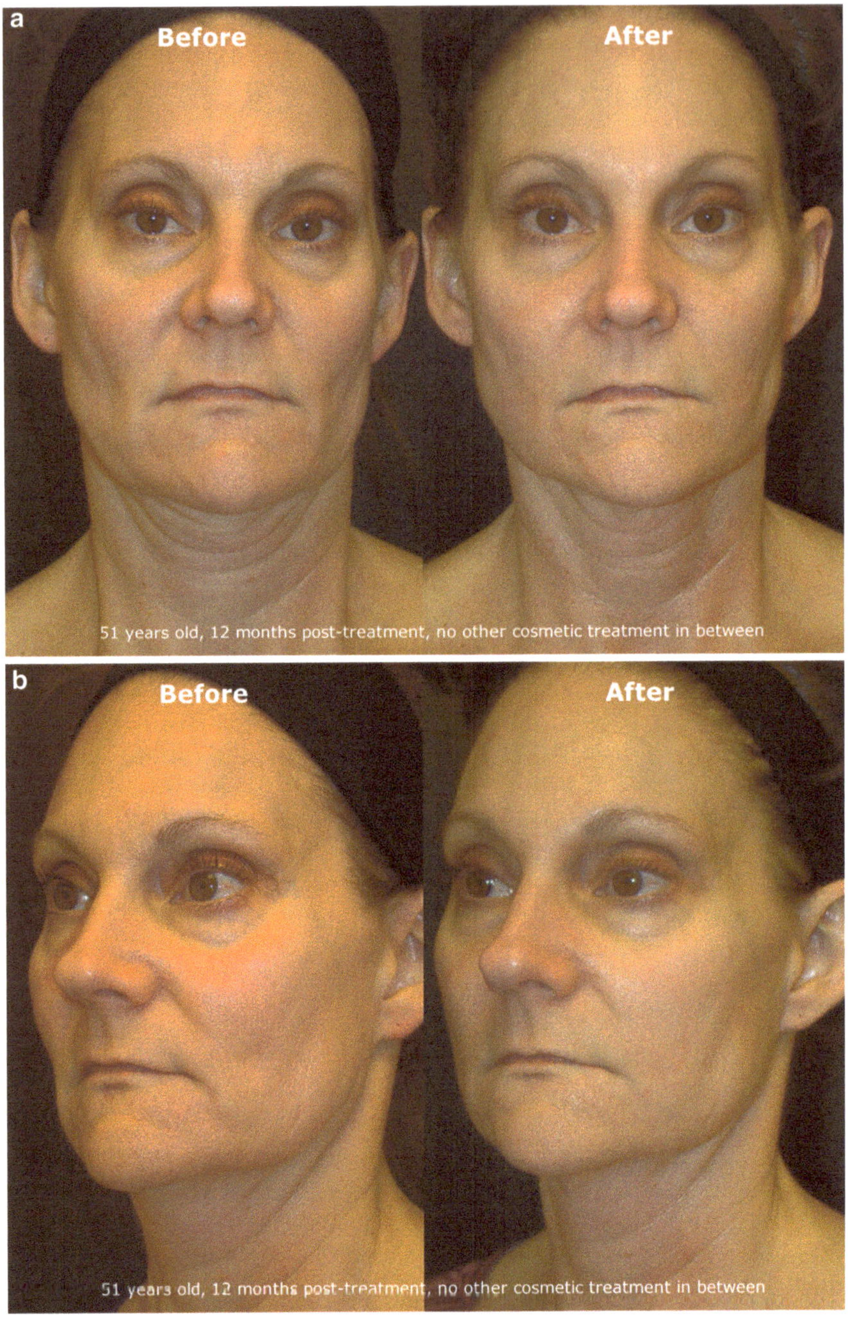


**Fig. 5.3** 51 years old, 12 months posttreatment, no other cosmetic treatment in between ((**a**) Front, (**b**) angled left, (**c**) left side, (**d**) angled right, (**e**) right side)

before the patient leaves the office. Ultherapy patients should be instructed that mild erythema may continue for a few days, but, if any other issues arise, to contact the physician. Most ultrasound or RF patients will be able to return to a full family, social, and work schedule immediately (barring the effects of any sedatives). Patients should be instructed to report any crusts, eschars, or blisters because they may be a sign of epidermal disruption from a burn. Those patients should return for

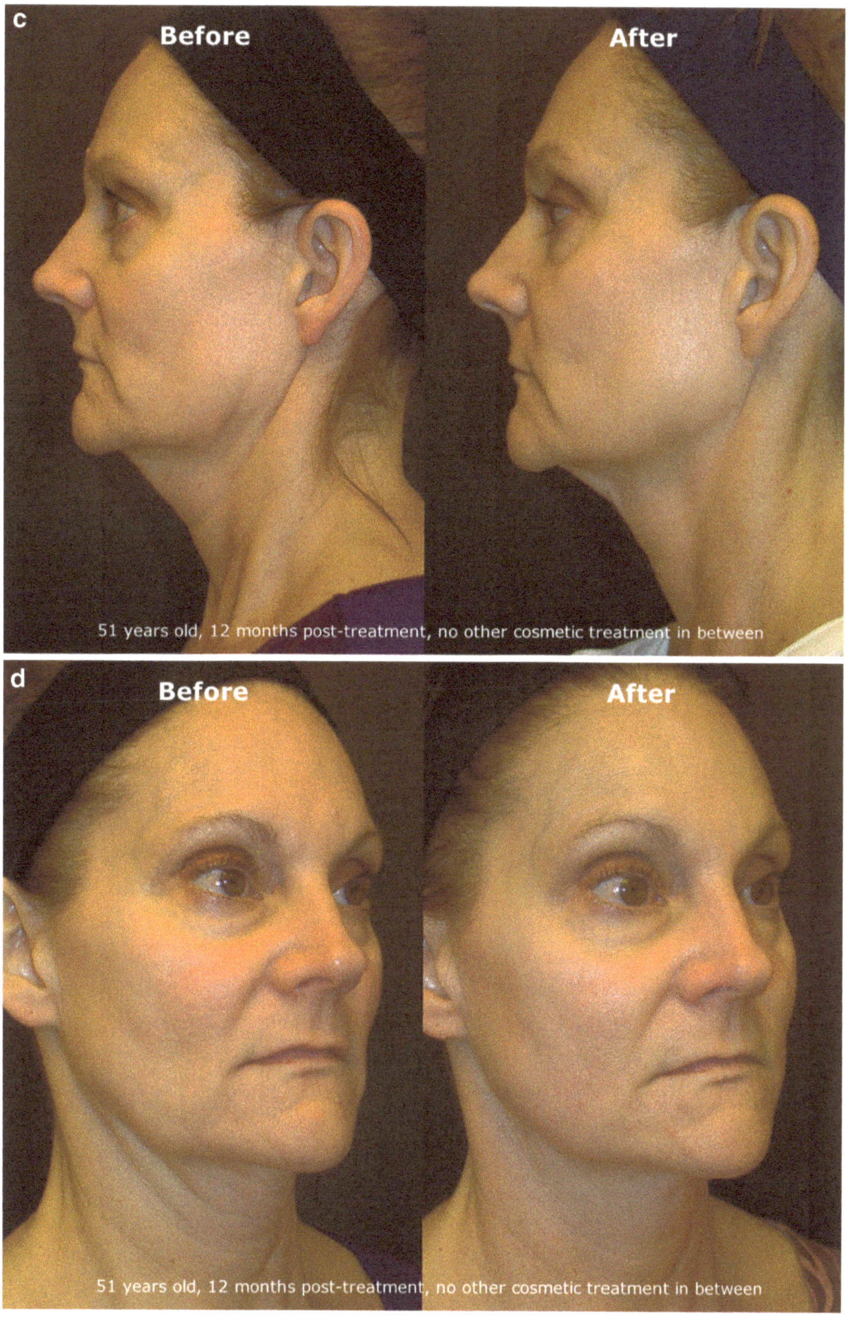


**Fig. 5.3** (continued)

evaluation and immediate treatment, with a moderate-potency topical corticosteroid and moist wound care with a bland ointment (petrolatum) prescribed. Often, blistering of mild burns can be avoided by evaluating the patient carefully before discharge. Focal areas of erythema and/or edema can be treated preventively with cold compresses and moderate-potency topical corticosteroids. Ice directly over the site should be avoided as this can result in further trauma to the skin.

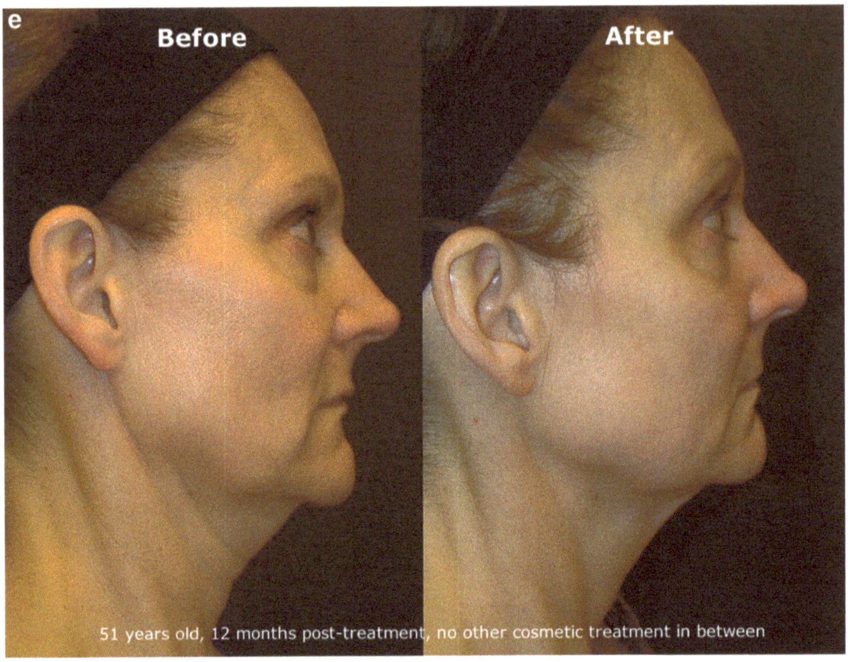


**Fig. 5.3** (continued)

Thermage patients treated using an eyeshield should be warned of the small risk of corneal abrasion during placement or removal. If the patient complains of a grainy sensation, erythromycin ophthalmic ointment is given. For persistent symptoms, patients should be referred for eye examination. Occasionally patients will note a "tingling" or sensitivity along bony areas like the brow or jawline for 24 h, but that has become uncommon with the newest protocols.

## Complications

First and foremost, training is the sine qua non of avoiding complications for both RF and ultrasound. Additionally, the maintenance and care of the device is extremely important as well. If in doubt about a patient or the device, it is best to postpone treatment. And despite excellent safety profiles, any device delivering heat to the skin must be used with caution. Always start with the "gentlest" treatment parameters when getting used to a new device and procedure.

### Radiofrequency

Certain preoperative measures can aid in avoiding complications. With Thermage, the primary complications are due to excessive heating. Thus, stacking consecutive pulses should be avoided. [58]. Patients must be instructed and then reminded to give feedback on discomfort. A scale of 0 ("I feel nothing") to 4 ("don't do that to me again") is easy to comprehend: if discomfort rises above a 2 ("I feel the heat but it is very tolerable"), depending on the degree, vibration and coupling fluid are increased and fluence can be reduced. If erythema is noted, move treatment to another area until clear. Excessive heating can result in blister and scar formation and, if pulses are stacked, delayed atrophy, particularly over bony prominences. Transient paresthesias of the jawline were commonplace with original versions of the device but are rare with the Thermage CPT system and current recommended moderate heat-multiple pulse protocol. Recent software upgrades have made it impossible to deliver pulses without adequate cryogen supply for cooling and the canister can be replaced during treatment. The device will provide warnings if the grounding pad is not properly connected. It is important to check the connection before continuing treatment. Finally, to avoid burning, adequate coupling fluid must be used and full contact with the treatment tip maintained.

Careful attention to details of the locations to be treated and the anatomical arrangement of the facial nerves is also important. Because heat is delivered deep enough to cause nerve irritation, herpes virus may be reactivated. Thus, antiviral prophylaxis for patients with any history of facial herpes simplex virus should be given the day of treatment. Oral antibiotics are unnecessary, because the epidermis remains intact. Treatment over subcutaneous acne nodules is not contraindicated, and results from handheld acne devices suggest the heat may actually reduce inflammation [69]. However treatment should not be performed over active infection or any non-intact skin.

While not a complication, inadequate results are a concern for patients. Because results are based on the patient's regenerative capabilities, younger patients with healthier skin will generally see more significant results. If patients are not pleased with the results, or if no significant improvements are noted photographically, retreating is generally not indicated. Patients pleased with the treatment who want additional improvement can be retreated after 6 months, although Dr. Waldorf generally suggests patients wait a year since additional tightening may be seen between 6 and 9 months.

## Ultrasound

As with radiofrequency, few complications exist with IUS. Immediately posttreatment, mild, transient erythema, edema, and swelling should be expected [15, 23, 32, 57, 67]. These usually diminish within a week or two.

The most concerning potential complication of Ultrasound therapy is nerve damage, especially of the marginal mandibular nerve from excessive heat in that area which can lead to a temporary unilateral palsy. A thorough history can also determine any previous history of Bell's palsy, which could be reactivated or worsened by any of these procedures. It is important to pay particular attention to avoidance of the delivery of energy over nerve danger zones. With careful attention to technique, these are extremely rare but still may occur if there is an unusual anatomical arrangement of the nerve. In his practice, Dr. Schlessinger does not use antibiotics but does treat for herpes prophylaxis for susceptible individuals.

It is important to note that when using the 10 MHz with 1.5 mm focal depth probe, if the probe tilts so that it is not completely perpendicular with the plane of the skin, temporary striations/welts will likely occur. This is due to the very superficial nature of this probe. These striations may also occur when treating too deeply around bone.

Chan et al. reported moderate postinflammatory hyperpigmentation (PIH) in 2.9 % of treatment sessions in a study of IUS treatment with Asian skin. PIH occurred when patients were treated with the 7.5 MHz, 4.5 mm focal depth probe on the forehead, but was not accompanied by any other adverse events such as blistering, severe erythema, or edema. PIH improved over 6 months posttreatment and was completely diminished by 9 months posttreatment. The authors believe it may be due to reflection of the IUS on the forehead bone, causing small, 2 mm round areas of PIH [15]. In his practice, Dr. Schlessinger has not observed this and routinely treats patients with skin of color.

## Other Treatment Modalities

### Pellevé

Pellevé (Ellman International, Oceanside, NY) is a monopolar radiofrequency device designed to treat mild to moderate skin laxity and early signs of aging. It was cleared by the FDA in 2009 for the treatment of mild to moderate facial wrinkles skin types I to IV with a duration claim of 6 months. It differs from other monopolar radiofrequency devices such as Thermage in that heating occurs gradually, so the skin becomes more accustomed to the heat changes. This means that no anesthesia has been needed in its studies, but some patients may still prefer a modest amount of anesthetic whether in the form of oral medication, vibration, or cooling. Patients should be informed that, although some improvement will be seen with the first session, multiple treatments are necessary to see full results generally at 2–4-week intervals. Additionally, since this procedure is radiofrequency and does not target melanocytes, it is also "color-blind" like Thermage [70, 71].

Rusciani et al. treated 93 patients (83 female, 10 male, mean age 53.3) with a single pass of radiofrequency over the full face. No anesthesia was given. Side effects included erythema, which lasted for 4–6 h. An initial contraction was noted, which lasted for 48–72 h. Blinded investigators rated an average improvement of 42.5 % after 1 month posttreatment, 37.5 % after 3 months, and 30 % after 6 months. 87 % of patients maintained results after 6 months [70, 71].

## Exilis

Exilis (BTL, Boston, MA) is another monopolar radiofrequency device designed to treat mild to moderate skin laxity and early signs of aging. It was cleared by the FDA in 2009 for the noninvasive treatment of wrinkles and rhytides [72]. It differs from other monopolar radiofrequency devices in that the device monitors the energy output levels and keeps them relatively constant. When an energy spike occurs, the device automatically reduces energy output. This is called the energy flow control system. Additionally, if the device senses poor skin contact, it shuts off the energy. These two features are said to ensure additional safety and reduce the chance of burns. The Exilis has platform options for face or body treatment and the benefit of not requiring disposables.

At the time this chapter was written, there were no peer-reviewed, indexed articles about Exilis. This is often the case with newer technologies, and the authors hope there will be more literature available shortly.

## References


1. 15th Annual Cosmetic Surgery National Data Bank Statistics. The American Society for Aesthetic Plastic Surgery, 2011.
2. 2011 AAFPRS Membership Study. American Academy of Facial Plastic and Reconstructive Surgery, 2011.
3. Alster TS, Lupton JR. Nonablative cutaneous remodeling using radiofrequency devices. Clin Dermatol. 2007;25(5):487–91.
4. Dierickx CC. The role of deep heating for noninvasive skin rejuvenation. Lasers Surg Med. 2006;38(9):799–807.
5. Alam M. Cosmetic dermatology for skin of color. New York: McGraw-Hill Medical; 2009. 186 p.
6. Bäck LJJ, Hytönen ML, Roine RP, Malmivaara AOV. Radiofrequency ablation treatment of soft palate for patients with snoring: a systematic review of effectiveness and adverse effects. Laryngoscope. 2009;119(6):1241–50.
7. Blumen MB, Dahan S, Fleury B, Hausser-Hauw C, Chabolle F. Radiofrequency ablation for the treatment of mild to moderate obstructive sleep apnea. Laryngoscope. 2002;112(11):2086–92.
8. Casal RF, Tam AL, Eapen GA. Radiofrequency ablation of lung tumors. Clin Chest Med. 2010;31(1):151–63; Table of Contents.
9. Dib RE, Touma NJ, Kapoor A. Review of the efficacy and safety of radiofrequency ablation for the treatment of small renal masses. Can Urol Assoc J. 2009;3(2):143–9.
10. Sutherland LM, Williams JA, Padbury RT, Gotley DC, Stokes B, Maddern GJ. Radiofrequency ablation of liver tumors: a systematic review. Arch Surg. 2006;141(2):181–90.
11. Wiesfeld ACP, Tan ES, Van Veldhuisen DJ, Crijns HJGM, Van Gelder IC. Radiofrequency ablation of atrial fibrillation. Int J Cardiol. 2004;93(2–3):231–7.
12. Chaudhari M. Radiofrequency techniques in pain management. Anaesth Intensive Care Med. 2011;12(2):63–5.
13. Alexiades-Armenakas M, Dover JS, Arndt KA. Unipolar versus bipolar radiofrequency treatment of rhytides and laxity using a mobile painless delivery method. Lasers Surg Med. 2008;40(7):446–53.
14. Lolis MS, Goldberg DJ. Radiofrequency in cosmetic dermatology: a review. Dermatol Surg. 2012;38(11):1765–76.
15. Chan NPY, Shek SYN, Yu CS, Ho SGY, Yeung CK, Chan HHL. Safety study of transcutaneous focused ultrasound for non-invasive skin tightening in Asians. Lasers Surg Med. 2011;43(5):366–75.
16. Sukal SA, Geronemus RG. Thermage: the nonablative radiofrequency for rejuvenation. Clin Dermatol. 2008;26(6):602–7. Epub 2008/10/23.
17. Wu WT. Achieving optimal results with thermage using mesoanesthesia and revised treatment parameters. Aesthet Surg J. 2007;27(1):93–9. Epub 2007/01/01.

18. Zelickson BD, Kist D, Bernstein E, Brown DB, Ksenzenko S, Burns J, et al. Histological and ultrastructural evaluation of the effects of a radiofrequency-based nonablative dermal remodeling device: a pilot study. Arch Dermatol. 2004;140(2):204–9. Epub 2004/02/18.
19. Polder KD, Bruce S. Radiofrequency: thermage. Facial Plast Surg Clin North Am. 2011;19(2):347–59. Epub 2011/07/19.
20. Kleinerman R, Whang TB, Bard RL, Marmur ES. Ultrasound in dermatology: principles and applications. J Am Acad Dermatol. 2012;67(3):478–87.
21. Email interview with Michael Floegel. 2010.
22. Suh DH, Chang KY, Son HC, Ryu JH, Lee SJ, Song KY. Radiofrequency and 585-nm pulsed dye laser treatment of striae distensae: a report of 37 Asian patients. Dermatol Surg. 2007;33(1):29–34. Epub 2007/01/12.
23. Suh DH, Shin MK, Lee SJ, Rho JH, Lee MH, Kim NI, et al. Intense focused ultrasound tightening in asian skin: clinical and pathologic results. Dermatol Surg. 2011;37(11):1595–602.
24. Elsaie ML, Choudhary S, Leiva A, Nouri K. Nonablative radiofrequency for skin rejuvenation. Dermatol Surg. 2010;36(5):577–89. Epub 2010/04/14.
25. Ruiz-Esparza J. Nonablative radiofrequency for facial and neck rejuvenation. A faster, safer, and less painful procedure based on concentrating the heat in key areas: the ThermaLift concept. J Cosmet Dermatol. 2006;5(1):68–75.
26. Anolik R, Chapas AM, Brightman LA, Geronemus RG. Radiofrequency devices for body shaping: a review and study of 12 patients. Semin Cutan Med Surg. 2009;28(4):236–43. Epub 2010/02/04.
27. England LJ, Tan MH, Shumaker PR, Egbert BM, Pittelko K, Orentreich D, et al. Effects of monopolar radiofrequency treatment over soft-tissue fillers in an animal model. Lasers Surg Med. 2005;37(5):356–65. Epub 2005/10/22.
28. Goldman MP, Alster TS, Weiss R. A randomized trial to determine the influence of laser therapy, monopolar radiofrequency treatment, and intense pulsed light therapy administered immediately after hyaluronic acid gel implantation. Dermatol Surg. 2007;33(5):535–42. Epub 2007/04/25.
29. Shumaker PR, England LJ, Dover JS, Ross EV, Harford R, DeRienzo D, et al. Effect of monopolar radiofrequency treatment over soft-tissue fillers in an animal model: part 2. Lasers Surg Med. 2006;38(3):211–7.
30. Thermage Treatment Reference Guide. Hayward, CA: Solta Medical; 2010. p. 1–37.
31. Alam M, White LE, Martin N, Witherspoon J, Yoo S, West DP. Ultrasound tightening of facial and neck skin: a rater-blinded prospective cohort study. J Am Acad Dermatol. 2010;62(2):262–9. Epub 2010/02/02.
32. Alster TS, Tanzi EL. Noninvasive lifting of arm, thigh, and knee skin with transcutaneous intense focused ultrasound. Dermatol Surg. 2012;38(5):754–9.
33. Burns AJ, Holden SG. Monopolar radiofrequency tissue tightening—how we do it in our practice. Lasers Surg Med. 2006;38(6):575–9.
34. Weiss RA, Weiss MA, Beasley KL, Munavalli G. Our approach to non-ablative treatment of photoaging. Lasers Surg Med. 2005;37(1):2–8. Epub 2005/07/22.
35. Atiyeh B, Dibo S. Nonsurgical nonablative treatment of aging skin: radiofrequency technologies between aggressive marketing and evidence-based efficacy. Aesthetic Plast Surg. 2009;33(3):283–94.
36. Helfrich YR, Sachs DL, Voorhees JJ. Overview of skin aging and photoaging. Dermatol Nurs. 2008;20(3):177–83; quiz 84. Epub 2008/07/25.
37. Burns JA. Thermage: monopolar radiofrequency. Aesthet Surg J. 2005;25(6):638–42. Epub 2005/11/01.
38. Pope K, Levinson M, Ross EV. Selective fibrous septae heating: an additional mechanism of action for capacitively coupled monopolar radiofrequency. Hayward, CA: Thermage, Inc.; 2005.
39. Hsu TS, Kaminer MS. The use of nonablative radiofrequency technology to tighten the lower face and neck. Semin Cutan Med Surg. 2003;22(2):115–23. Epub 2003/07/25.
40. White WM, Makin IR, Slayton MH, Barthe PG, Gliklich R. Selective transcutaneous delivery of energy to porcine soft tissues using intense ultrasound (IUS). Lasers Surg Med. 2008;40(2):67–75. Epub 2008/02/29.
41. Hruza GJ. Rejuvenating the aging face. Arch Facial Plast Surg. 2004;6(6):366–9. Epub 2004/11/17.
42. Kim KH, Geronemus RG. Nonablative laser and light therapies for skin rejuvenation. Arch Facial Plast Surg. 2004;6(6):398–409. Epub 2004/11/17.
43. Kirsch KM, Zelickson BD, Zachary CB, Tope WD. Ultrastructure of collagen thermally denatured by microsecond domain pulsed carbon dioxide laser. Arch Dermatol. 1998;134(10):1255–9. Epub 1998/11/05.
44. Ross EV, Naseef GS, McKinlay JR, Barnette DJ, Skrobal M, Grevelink J, et al. Comparison of carbon dioxide laser, erbium:YAG laser, dermabrasion, and dermatome: a study of thermal damage, wound contraction, and wound healing in a live pig model: implications for skin resurfacing. J Am Acad Dermatol. 2000;42(1 Pt 1):92–105. Epub 1999/12/22.
45. Fitzpatrick R, Geronemus R, Goldberg D, Kaminer M, Kilmer S, Ruiz-Esparza J. Multicenter study of noninvasive radiofrequency for periorbital tissue tightening. Lasers Surg Med. 2003;33(4):232–42. Epub 2003/10/23.
46. Narins DJ, Narins RS. Non-surgical radiofrequency facelift. J Drugs Dermatol. 2003;2(5):495–500. Epub 2003/10/16.
47. Alster TS, Tanzi E. Improvement of neck and cheek laxity with a nonablative radiofrequency device: a lifting experience. Dermatol Surg. 2004;30(4 Pt 1):503–7; discussion 7. Epub 2004/04/02.
48. Bassichis BA, Dayan S, Thomas JR. Use of a nonablative radiofrequency device to rejuvenate the upper one-third of the face. Otolaryngol Head Neck Surg. 2004;130(4):397–406.

49. Fritz M, Counters JT, Zelickson BD. Radiofrequency treatment for middle and lower face laxity. Arch Facial Plast Surg. 2004;6(6):370–3. Epub 2004/11/17.
50. Laubach HJ, Makin IR, Barthe PG, Slayton MH, Manstein D. Intense focused ultrasound: evaluation of a new treatment modality for precise microcoagulation within the skin. Dermatol Surg. 2008;34(5):727–34. Epub 2008/04/24.
51. White WM, Makin IR, Barthe PG, Slayton MH, Gliklich RE. Selective creation of thermal injury zones in the superficial musculoaponeurotic system using intense ultrasound therapy: a new target for noninvasive facial rejuvenation. Arch Facial Plast Surg. 2007;9(1):22–9. Epub 2007/01/17.
52. Fatemi A. High-intensity focused ultrasound effectively reduces adipose tissue. Semin Cutan Med Surg. 2009;28(4):257–62. Epub 2010/02/04.
53. Fatemi A, Kane MA. High-intensity focused ultrasound effectively reduces waist circumference by ablating adipose tissue from the abdomen and flanks: a retrospective case series. Aesthetic Plast Surg. 2010;34(5):577–82. Epub 2010/04/13.
54. Gadsden E, Aguilar MT, Smoller BR, Jewell ML. Evaluation of a novel high-intensity focused ultrasound device for ablating subcutaneous adipose tissue for noninvasive body contouring. Aesthet Surg J. 2011;31(4):401–10.
55. Jewell ML, Desilets C, Smoller BR. Evaluation of a novel high-intensity focused ultrasound device. Aesthet Surg J. 2011;31(4):429–34.
56. Jewell ML, Weiss RA, Baxter RA, Cox SE, Dover JS, Donofrio LM, et al. Safety and tolerability of high-intensity focused ultrasonography for noninvasive body sculpting: 24-week data from a randomized, sham-controlled study. Aesthet Surg J. 2012;32(7):868–76. Epub 2012/09/04.
57. Lee HS, Jang WS, Cha Y-J, Choi Y-H, Tak Y, Hwang E, et al. Multiple pass ultrasound tightening of skin laxity of the lower face and neck. Dermatol Surg. 2012;38(1):20–7.
58. Narins RS, Tope WD, Pope K, Ross EV. Overtreatment effects associated with a radiofrequency tissue tightening device: rare, preventable, and correctable with subcision and autologous fat transfer. Dermatol Surg. 2006;32(1):115–24.
59. Abraham MT, Chiang SK, Keller GS, Rawnsley JD, Blackwell KE, Elashoff DA. Clinical evaluation of non-ablative radiofrequency facial rejuvenation. J Cosmet Laser Ther. 2004;6(3):136–44. Epub 2004/11/17.
60. Melzack R, Wall PD. Pain mechanisms: a new theory. Science. 1965;150(3699):971–9. Epub 1965/11/19.
61. Binder A, Baron R. Utility of transcutaneous electrical nerve stimulation in neurologic pain disorders. Neurology. 2010;74(2):104–5. Epub 2010/01/01.
62. Dubinsky RM, Miyasaki J. Assessment: efficacy of transcutaneous electric nerve stimulation in the treatment of pain in neurologic disorders (an evidence-based review): report of the Therapeutics and Technology Assessment Subcommittee of the American Academy of Neurology. Neurology. 2010; 74(2):173–6. Epub 2010/01/01.
63. Vibration therapy for pain. Lancet. 1992;339(8808): 1513–4. Epub 1992/06/20.
64. Smith KC, Comite SL, Balasubramanian S, Carver A, Liu JF. Vibration anesthesia: a noninvasive method of reducing discomfort prior to dermatologic procedures. Dermatol Online J. 2004;10(2):1. Epub 2004/11/09.
65. Alam M, Levy R, Pajvani U, Ramierez JA, Guitart J, Veen H, et al. Safety of radiofrequency treatment over human skin previously injected with medium-term injectable soft-tissue augmentation materials: a controlled pilot trial. Lasers Surg Med. 2006;38(3):205–10. Epub 2006/03/15.
66. Weiss RA, Weiss MA, Munavalli G, Beasley KL. Monopolar radiofrequency facial tightening: a retrospective analysis of efficacy and safety in over 600 treatments. J Drugs Dermatol. 2006;5(8):707–12. Epub 2006/09/23.
67. Gliklich RE, White WM, Slayton MH, Barthe PG, Makin IR. Clinical pilot study of intense ultrasound therapy to deep dermal facial skin and subcutaneous tissues. Arch Facial Plast Surg. 2007;9(2):88–95. Epub 2007/03/21.
68. Phone interview with Dr. Thomas Hitchcock. 2012.
69. Badgwell Doherty C, Doherty SD, Rosen T. Thermotherapy in dermatologic infections. J Am Acad Dermatol. 2010;62(6):909–27; quiz 28. Epub 2010/05/15.
70. Rusciani A, Curinga G, Menichini G, Alfano C, Rusciani L. Nonsurgical tightening of skin laxity: a new radiofrequency approach. J Drugs Dermatol. 2007;6(4):381–6. Epub 2007/08/03.
71. Stampar M. The Pelleve procedure: an effective method for facial wrinkle reduction and skin tightening. Facial Plast Surg Clin North Am. 2011;19(2):335–45.
72. Section 5 - 510(k) Summary For EXILIS. In: DHHS, editor. 2009. p. 6.

# Filler Augmentation

# 6

Steven H. Dayan, Tara E. Brennan,
and John P. Arkins

## Introduction to Different Fillers for the Periorbital, Forehead, and Midface

The importance of the appearance of the periorbital region is imperative in the analysis of facial aesthetics because of the inordinate amount of relevant information it subconsciously transmits. The eyes can signal female sexual arousal [1, 2], fertility [3], and aggression [4] and have evolved to be the first site of inspection [5], an innate instinct devoid of social imprinting and present even among infants [6]. Hence, it is reasonable to conclude that one's first impressions are heavily influenced by the impression of the upper and midfacial region [7].

Improving the aesthetic appearance of this region, therefore, has potential to influence one's evaluation by others, and multiple studies have shown that more favorable first impressions are made after split-second exposure to photos of persons who have undergone mid- and upper facial rejuvenation procedures [8–11]. Furthermore, it has been shown that minimally invasive cosmetic procedures to the upper and midface result in improvements to one's self-esteem and quality of life [10, 12].

These important improvements are aimed at mitigating the effects of aging on the upper and midface. The effects of aging on the periorbital and midfacial regions are a result of a combination of factors, including the effects of gravity, sun exposure, reduction in skin thickness, and volume loss [13]. The deleterious effects of smoking, too, cannot be overemphasized and include impaired wound healing, characteristic perioral as well as overall facial skin wrinkling, and a generally accelerated process of skin aging [14, 15]. A youthful and beautiful female face draws attention to the eyes and assumes an inverted triangle with its greatest width at the cheeks and driving to a narrow point at the chin. Moreover, the preference for females with high cheekbones, large eyes, and a small chin is evolutionarily preserved across both developed and tribal cultures around the world [16]. However, as

Electronic supplementary material The online version of this chapter (doi:10.1007/978-1-4614-8388-5_6) contains supplementary material, which is available to authorized users.

S.H. Dayan, M.D., F.A.C.S. (✉)
Chicago Center for Facial Plastic Surgery,
845 North Michigan Avenue, Suite 923E,
Chicago, IL 60611, USA

DeNova Research, Chicago, IL, USA

Department of Otolaryngology-Head
and Neck Surgery, University of Illinois at Chicago,
Chicago, IL, USA

School of New Learning, DePaul University,
Chicago, IL, USA
e-mail: sdayan@drdayan.com

T.E. Brennan, M.D.
Department of Otolaryngology-Head
and Neck Surgery, University of Illinois at Chicago,
Chicago, IL, USA

J.P. Arkins, B.S.
DeNova Research, Chicago, IL, USA

S.A. Myint (ed.), *Nonsurgical Peri-orbital Rejuvenation*, DOI 10.1007/978-1-4614-8388-5_6,

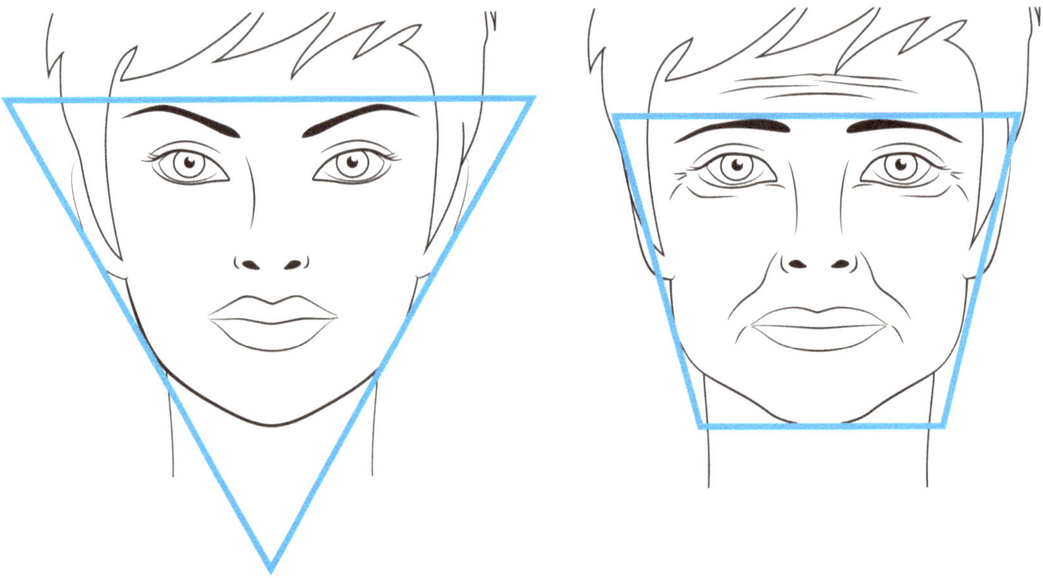

**Fig. 6.1** A youthful female face is representative of an *upside-down triangle*, whereas an aged face descends over time and the chin becomes more *square-like*

a female ages, the cheeks descend to create a hollowing effect around the eyes. As the malar fat pad descends over the jawline, "jowling" occurs, which results in the chin appearing square-like, as opposed to an upside-down triangle female (Fig. 6.1). This downward descent has a masculinizing effect on the aging female [17].

It follows, therefore, that much attention has been focused among aesthetic facial surgeons on the task of periorbital rejuvenation. Historically, upper and midfacial rejuvenation has included surgical interventions like rhytidectomy and blepharoplasty to mitigate the long-term effects of gravity. Specifically, the orbitomalar ligament develops laxity with age, which leads to inferior descent of the suborbicularis oculi fat and skeletonization of the inferior orbital rim [18]. An extended blepharoplasty works by resuspending the orbitomalar ligament and suborbicularis oculi fat to achieve midfacial elevation [19]. Similarly, a facelift works by resuspending downwardly displaced submuscular aponeurotic tissue and trimming excess, thinned overlying skin. This redraping of tightened skin reduces the "sagging" effects of age.

More recently, there has been a trend towards less invasive dermatologic rejuvenation interventions in order to improve the aesthetics of the face in this region. The popularity of soft tissue fillers, in particular, has increased 190 % in the last 10 years [20] due in large part to the less invasive nature of these procedures as compared to their traditional surgical counterparts. Likewise, these minimally invasive procedures carry with them less inconvenience, recovery time, overall expense, and fewer overall risks, including the elimination of risks imposed by general anesthesia.

Restoration of volume loss can be achieved with placement of syringe-based fillers, autologous fat, or implants. By placing a soft tissue filler in the cheeks and infraorbital areas, fillers can be used to mitigate lower eyelid contour defects, raise the cheek lid pedestal, and rejuvenate the brows—in essence, framing the eyes. Patients who lack significant volume loss and who do not require lower lid blepharoplasty to address periorbital aging concerns may be candidates for office-based volume replacement using syringe-based fillers. Those with more severe volume loss or those who would require multiple syringes of filler to achieve desired results may be better candidates for autologous fat injection, which has the advantage of being more durable and with potentially longer-term graft survival, but the disadvantage of additional donor site morbidity, albeit minor, and surgical time [21].

Broadly, facial fillers can be divided into four categories: hyaluronic acid, synthetic fillers, autologous fat, and collagens. They may also be divided based on the depth of their injection: subdermal (i.e., calcium hydroxylapatite, or Radiesse) versus intradermal (hyaluronic acid, or Restylane, Perlane, or Juvéderm) [22]. It is the senior author's experience that each filler has unique physical properties that lend to specific outcomes in individual patients. It is paramount to consider the unique physical properties prior to deciding which filler is best for the patient.

## Hyaluronic Acid

Hyaluronic acid (HA) is a collagen replacement product that comes in a variety of chemically similar but structurally different forms. HA is a naturally occurring glycosaminoglycan that is a major component of all connective tissue and exhibits no species or tissue specificity [22]. HA is a nonanimal product, and thus, there is no potential for an adverse immunologic reaction to HA. Therefore, no preinjection allergic testing is required. In addition, HA plays an important role in dermal hydration; decreases in HA with age result in reduced dermal thickness, increased skin wrinkling, and folding.

HAs are the most popular soft tissue filler in the United States and comprised 85 % of filler treatments in 2010 [23]. Restylane/Perlane (Medicis Aesthetics, Scottsdale, AZ) and Juvéderm Ultra/Ultraplus (Allergan, Irvine, CA) are the most popular HA products used as effective dermal fillers for cosmetic and reconstructive purposes. Patients who lack a severe degree of aging-associated facial volume loss may be candidates for HA injection. In addition, HA can be reversed within 12–24 h following injection of hyaluronidase. Juvéderm is FDA approved for 12 months on initial treatment and 18 months with retreatment for Restylane. However, anecdotally, both HAs can persist well beyond a year with documented occurrences of Restylane persisting for 5 years [24]. A 2007 report demonstrated that HA can stimulate collagen production [25] and perhaps this contributes to its extended correction. If placed in large quantities or if an early retreatment is given, the product seems to last longer and can persist at 36 months [26]. However, while the currently marketed soft tissue fillers are often thought of interchangeably, each HA has unique properties that should be considered when evaluating candidates for injection [27].

Juvéderm is marketed as the "smoother filler" with a gel-like 24 mg/mL concentration of HA and hydrophilic properties six times that of Restylane [28]. In contrast, Restylane is over six times more resistant to deformation than Juvéderm as defined by its rheological properties G' [28]. It is the differences between Restylane and Juvéderm that the senior author frequently relies upon when selecting an HA for a specific indication. Juvéderm-corrected areas tend to lead to a fuller and more diffuse augmentation as water is absorbed. Moreover, the results of Juvéderm augmentation are more likely to be affected by the body's current level of hydration. Consequently, knowledge of its greater hydrophilicity should be considered when injecting. In particular, Juvéderm, with its highly hydrophilic nature, tends to attract more fluid and, therefore, results in a diffuse filling effect.

For the buccal cheek space, the diffuse filling properties inherent to Juvéderm have shown to be more beneficial. However, in the infraorbital tear trough, Restylane is preferred. The differences between Restylane and Juvéderm are extremely apparent when placed into the loose areolar tissues surrounding the orbital region. When treating this area, the senior author prefers Restylane to Juvéderm as the latter will attract water, swell, and result in dark puffy under-eye circles representative of a tired unflattering appearance. While this can occur with both Juvéderm and Restylane when placed under the eyes, it—the Tyndall effect, in which the optical chamber of HA and fluid reflects blue light—is more commonly associated with Juvéderm. In patients with thin, translucent skin, the blueness is distracting and obvious.

Perlane and Juvéderm Ultraplus are HA products of a larger particle size. While both Perlane and Juvéderm Ultraplus are at the same concentration of HA as their smaller particle-sized counterparts, the large particle size provides a more robust alternative intended for deeper placement into the soft tissues with potential for greater product longevity [29]. However, clinically appreciable differences are not as apparent and rarely offset the greater cost of the product.

In addition to the current HA fillers available, the large particle Allergan Voluma and Restylane SubQ offer potential advances in facial shaping. Additionally, Belotero (Merz Aesthetics, San Mateo, CA) is a smooth consistency monophasic HA and is reported to provide correction without risk for a Tyndall effect due to its trademark cohesive polydensified matrix properties. This may prove to be a superior product for treating the tear trough.

## Synthetic Fillers

In contrast to the HA products previously discussed, Radiesse (Merz Aesthetics, San Mateo, CA) is a synthetic injectable implant composed of smooth calcium hydroxylapatite (CaHA) microspheres suspended in a sodium carboxymethylcellulose gel carrier. It is a more substantial facial filler than HA and thus tends to be more effective in treating more deep lines and furrows [30]. The body slowly degrades the CaHA microspheres after injection, whose treatment effect is estimated to last between 6 and 12 months. It is FDA approved for the correction of moderate to severe facial folds and wrinkles, as well as lipodystrophy. Like the HA products previously described, Radiesse does not contain animal products, so no allergic testing is required prior to its use. CaHA is particularly useful in highlighting bony prominences such as the malar area in patients with thicker skin. In contrast to HAs, CaHA has minimal hydrophilic properties and it is important to avoid placing the filler thinly or diffusely. CaHA is metabolized by enzymatic breakdown with absorption of microspheres evident at 9 months [31]. The senior author has experienced CaHA to predictably and routinely persist from nine to 12 months, regardless of the patient.

Poly-L-lactic acid (Sculptra, Sanofi Aventis, Bridgewater, NJ) is a product that relies on its controlled foreign body biostimulatory properties and is preferred by many physicians and patients for its subtle and progressive augmentation. However, too robust of a response can be problematic, resulting in nodules and, rarely, granulomas [32]. This product is primarily for patients requesting global facial volumization where autologous fat is not available. Poly-L-lactic acid is likely degraded by hydrolysis and extracellular enzymes and subsequently broken down by macrophages [31]. It can be expected to last from 12 to 18 months following a series of three treatments.

Other fillers that are used less often include the permanent silicone (Silikon 1000 purified polydimethylsiloxane, Alcon Laboratories, Fort Worth, TX) and polymethylmethacrylate (PMMA) (Artefill, Suneva, San Diego, CA). The firm nature of these products is advantageous for filling in the fine rhytides of the upper lip, scars, and deep etched-in dermal rhytides, but are not appropriate in periorbital augmentation.

## Autologous Fat

Autologous fat is not generally used in the clinic setting, but is very effective when high volumes are required for volume registration and tends to have a more long-lasting effect than HA dermal fillers. Additionally, autologous fat transfer to the head and neck region has been recently linked with promising ancillary benefits in addition to volume restoration, including overlying skin rejuvenation. It is unclear at this time to what this regenerative effect may be attributed, although there is good evidence that the regenerative effect of adipose-derived mesenchymal stem cells is responsible [33].

## Collagen

Collagen (Zyderm, Inamed, Santa Barbara, CA) was the first FDA-approved bovine filler for cosmetic use and was injected into the deep dermis to fill in fine wrinkles. However, hypersensitivity testing and limited duration ultimately led to the demise of collagen when Restylane garnered FDA approval in 2003. There was a brief resurgence in collagen popularity with the June 2008 FDA approval for porcine-derived collagen product Evolence (Johnson & Johnson, New Brunswick, NJ). Skin testing was unnecessary and a 12-month cosmetically appealing correction of an NLF could be expected. Unfortunately, the product did not achieve its business objectives and was discontinued in 2009.

## Botulinum Toxin Type A

Botulinum toxin is commonly used as an adjunct therapy to soft tissue fillers and, as such, deserves special mention here. For example, after toxin is used to treat dynamic rhytids in the forehead region, fillers may be employed to address the static rhytids that remain. When soft tissue filler techniques, with or without concomitant neurotoxin therapy, are used judiciously, they can effect subtle yet drastic improvements in facial appearance.

Soft tissue fillers have an overall excellent patient safety profile. However, complications can and do occur, and as the number of patients treated with soft tissue fillers increases commensurate with the demand for more minimally invasive facial rejuvenation procedures, so will the number of complications. As such, it is important that physicians interested in providing this service to patients be adequately informed regarding injection techniques and, perhaps more importantly, principles of facial analysis guiding the decision whether or not to employ these techniques. And, if so, where to place such injections to affect a particular desired change.

## Preinjection Evaluation of the Patient

When evaluating a patient who presents for facial rejuvenation procedures, it is best to start the evaluation as you would in another patient encounter, namely, by taking a history and focusing on eliciting the patient's major concerns about their appearance. Particular attention should be paid to their general concerns about their face and any specific aspects of their appearance they would like altered. This may include anything from depressed scars to rosacea to apparently thinning lips to periorbital wrinkles. This is critical because what the clinician may perceive as being a major contributor to the patient's aging appearance may not, in fact, be bothersome to the patient. In achieving an outcome that is overall satisfying to the patient, it is paramount to target their primary concerns in your treatment plan [34].

Patients may also present with more general complaints of feeling or looking "older" and seek your opinion regarding procedures that may be helpful in improving their overall appearance. It is with these patients that a holistic approach to facial analysis is even more salient than among those presenting to address a single, specific concern. In taking a holistic approach to facial analysis, one has the ability to examine a patient for opportunities to "rejuvenate" the face by making minor changes to restore a more youthful appearance to the face. This is done by keeping the general effects of aging on the face in mind that have been previously mentioned—namely, increased tissue laxity, "sagging," and (dermal and fat) volume loss [18]. To this effect, minor changes using a combination of neurotoxin and fillers can have subtle yet noticeably positive effects on patients.

Dayan and Arkins presented a case of a 37-year-old otherwise healthy Caucasian female who presented for evaluation desiring a more youthful appearance (Fig. 6.2a, b) [17]. Facial analysis was significant for mild malar volume loss and moderate forehead, glabellar, and periorbital rhytids. Following the philosophy that one's attention is drawn first to the eyes, attention was paid to this region. Specifically, volume was restored to the periorbital and malar areas using HA, resulting in the appearance of an inverted, and less square-like, orientation of the face. This created a more overall youthful feminine look. A combination of onabotulinumtoxinA and soft tissue filler was used to treat rhytids in the forehead/temple area. Details of the technique of this injection may be found in the next section of the chapter.

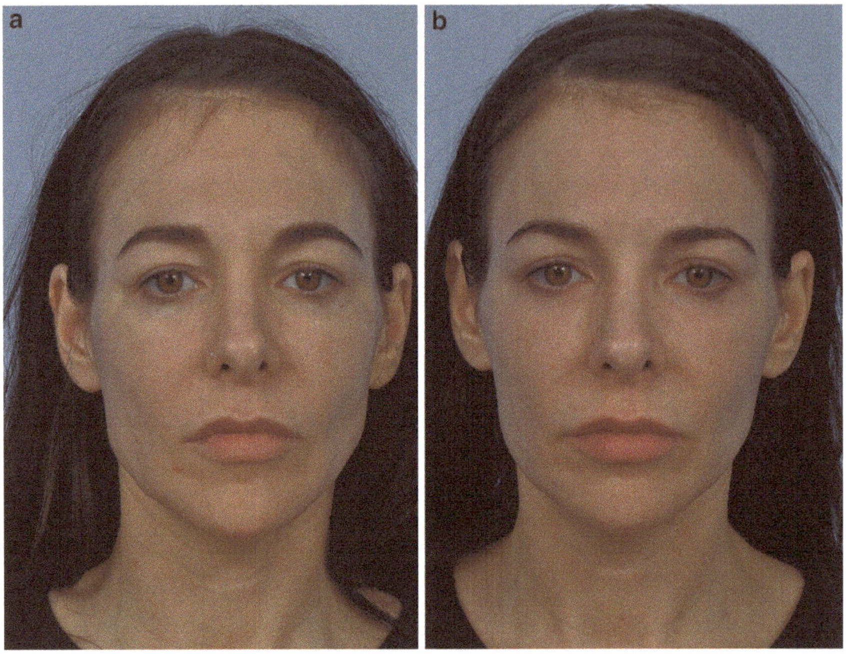

**Fig. 6.2** (**a**) A 37-year-old female prior to periorbital rejuvenation. (**b**) Improvement in facial volume loss and a decrease in rhytids noted at 2-week posttreatment

## Injection Techniques

One of the most important aspects to periorbital rejuvenation is more rooted in the ability to understand what makes someone *feel* attractive. This analysis is often more important than the selection of a particular product and one's injection technique. It is imperative to understand that at its core, beauty can serve as a subliminal indicator of our evolutionary fitness that is used to depict our health and vitality. Neural pathways in the posterior cingulated cortex and amygdala process facial characteristics [35] and determine an emotional response that allows humans to make personality judgments [35–37] within 39–100 ms [36, 37].

Moreover, an essential element to any cosmetic enhancement is that the alteration must appear natural and remain in the subconscious. Once elevated to the realm of the conscious, the pleasure-eliciting effects of beauty are greatly diminished [38]. The slightest evidence of cosmetic alteration can tip off the primitive subconscious that something has been done and that a possible genetic weakness may exist under the façade. It is the same reason that women are perceived more favorably when makeup is placed in moderation and more negatively when placed in excess [39].

As previously discussed, the eyes are the feature that is most commonly examined first [5, 40]. However, historically, periorbital rejuvenation has not been a primary focus when treating with soft tissue fillers. Likely driven by its FDA indications, soft tissue fillers have long been used in the treatment of the nasolabial fold region. However, augmenting treating this region is not always advisable. Filling the nasolabial fold augments and draws more attention to the lower third of the face. This may result in the chin appearing larger and the jaw appearing more square-like. It is the senior author's opinion that this visual effect is masculinizing—even simian-like—and should be avoided among females. In contrast, applying fillers to the upper and middle thirds has the ability to feminize the face through mitigation of lower eyelid contour defects, raising the cheek lid pedestal, and rejuvenating the brows. In doing so, one may directly address the atrophy, fat loss, and skeletal changes brought on by the aging process with filler augmentation.

When treating the periorbital region, one should attempt to make the eyes appear as large as possible—in part because the more childlike the eyes appear, the more attractive a female's face is perceived. Infantile eyes are large, light colored, and slightly further apart than those of an adult. A lateral outside corner of the eye that lies 2 mm above the inside corner of the eye is also considered highly attractive. In addition to this slight slant, eyes that are farther apart have been shown to be more attractive, regardless of culture [41].

In addition to treating within the larger context of subliminally influenced beauty, the use of blunt-tip cannulas instead of needles for injecting fillers allows for immediate results with minimal morbidity. Using the cannulas, the provider is able to place the fillers deep, resulting in a procedure that is less focused on the filling of superficial rhytids and is able to avoid the ecchymosis, discomfort, and edema often associated with treatments that are more superficial. Moreover, the cannulas allow the injector to dissect underlying soft tissue to select a precise plane for product placement. Importantly, using a blunt-tip cannula instead of a sharp needle in theory reduces the chance of inadvertent intravascular injection of filler, a disastrous complication.

It should be noted that there is a moderate learning curve to overcome when using the cannulas; however, thinning the filler with 1 % lidocaine increases the malleability of the product. Once placed, the filler can then be massaged into place. It should be noted that using a blunt-tip cannula requires more injecting force than its sharp needle-tip counterpart does. While the additional force required for a blunt-tip filler injection is not more painful, the increased pressure required may be initially unsettling to a patient who has had needle-tip injections in the past and is not advised of the difference with this injection technique.

The technique used in the treatment of the 37-year-old Caucasian female previously described is outlined here.

First, the face was cleansed with alcohol and betadine. Next, onabotulinumtoxinA (Botox Cosmetic, Irvine, CA) was reconstituted with bacteriostatic 2.2 cc of saline to create a final dilution of three units per 0.1 cc. The reconstituted onabotulinumtoxinA was then injected into the procerus, frontalis, corrugators, orbicularis oculi, and masseters (a total of 90 units). A blunt-tip cannula was used for this injection to assist in precise placement of filler product. Once the correct location and plane for filler placement is identified, the cannula is kept moving back and forth in a fanning fashion during a slow product injection. This assists in smooth and even deposition of product.

Next, HA, Restylane, was prepared. 2 mL of a 1 mL Restylane was added to 0.1 cc of saline and 0.1 cc of 1 % lidocaine. This mixture was injected into the temple area using a 22 gauge, 70 mm blunt-tip cannula. Next the malar areas were treated with 2 mL of a mixture of 1 mL of HA, 0.2 cc saline, and 0.1 cc 1 % lidocaine, again using a blunt-tip cannula. Following filler injection, the area was manually molded to ensure smooth and proper placement. This is important to avoid any unsightly lumping of product that will subsequently be felt (and seen) by the patient.

Another example involving subtle alterations using dermal fillers and botulinum toxin to produce a more upside-down triangle-oriented face that draws one's attention to the eyes is demonstrated, below (Fig. 6.3a–c). Here, a 30-year-old woman undergoes a series of treatment with onabotulinumtoxinA in the brow and masseters, CaHA fillers in the cheeks, and HA fillers in the lips, followed by fractionated $CO_2$ laser treatment. Additionally, the eyelashes were treated with bimatoprost, drawing further attention to the eyes on first glance. These photos were taken over the course of 19 months. Notably, the patient's weight remained constant during this time.

This example is significant because it demonstrates how the eyes and upper one-third of the face are emphasized while de-emphasizing the lower one-third, increasing the feminization of this patient's face. Specifically in this case, injecting neurotoxin into the masseter muscles narrows the jaw. In doing so, it also subtly draws attention to the lips, which were augmented using HA.

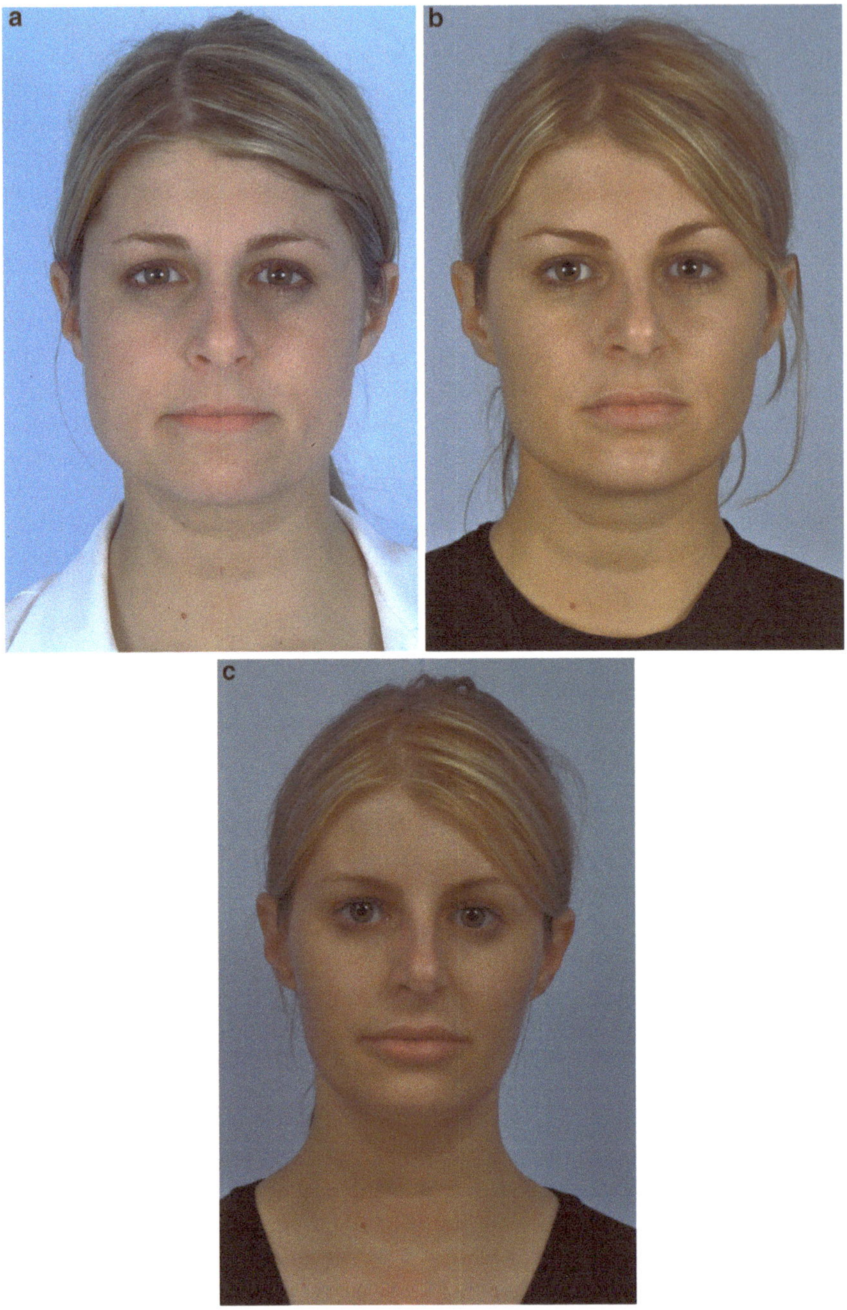

**Fig. 6.3** (**a**) Baseline, (**b**) 12-month, (**c**) and 18-month posttreatment of onabotulinumtoxinA, 0.03 % bimatoprost, and CaHA to the mid- and upper thirds

While women consistently make up about 90 % of plastic surgery patients, men are a growing segment that can benefit from periorbital soft tissue filler treatment. Interestingly, men and women differ when it comes to increasing the attractive appearance of the eyes. The more contrast apparent between the eyes and the surrounding skin and, consequently, the more attention drawn to the eyes, themselves, the more attractive a woman's eyes appear. However, a man with

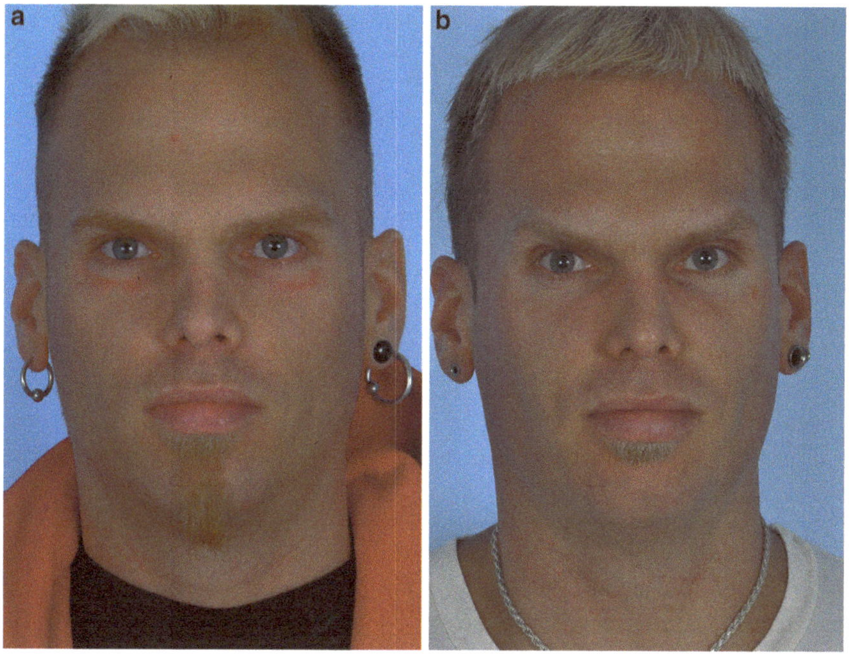

**Fig. 6.4** (**a**) Baseline (**b**) and 3 years post a series of treatments with onabotulinumtoxinA and poly-L-lactic acid to decrease the appearance of a heavy brow, frontal bone bossing, and facial hollows

dark eyes, particularly when deep set, may be seen as aggressive.

When treating male patients, the aesthetic provider should try to emphasize sexually dimorphic male traits while avoiding overemphasis of features that emphasize male dominance. Excessive dominance in facial features may be perceived negatively and threatening. An excessively broad chin, heavy brow, or darkened eyes may signal a man who is aggressive, dominant, unfriendly, threatening, volatile, controlling, manipulative, coercive, or selfish [42]. The dismissive attitude towards males with disproportionate facial dominant traits is likely due to the high testosterone levels in utero. Higher levels of testosterone are linked with dominance and competition and possibly violence [43]. Thus, it has become evolutionary adaptive to fear those with such physical traits [44].

A 42-year-old male hairdresser who felt that his facial appearance misrepresented his personality and detracted clients from his business presented with a heavy brow, frontal bone bossing, and facial hollows. A series of onabotulinumtoxinA (Botox Cosmetic, Allergan, Irvine, CA) treatments (30–45 units) over 3 years (12 total treatments) to his brow resulted in temporary reduction of anger animation and long-term atrophy of corrugator muscles. A series of poly-l-lactic acid (Sculptra, Sanofi Aventis, Bridgewater, NJ) injections over 2 years to fill in midfacial hollows and one treatment with one vial (1.0 cc) hyaluronic acid (Restylane, Medicis, Scottsdale, AZ) premixed with 0.3 cc of lidocaine with epinephrine placed via a 25 gauge 50 mm cannula (Merz Aesthetics, San Mateo, CA) to his forehead region camouflaged the frontal bone bossing (Fig. 6.4a–b).

## Postinjection Care and Follow-Up

In the experience of the senior author, minimal postinjection care, apart from application of an ice pack, is required. Postoperative antibiotics are not routinely administered. Patients may begin to see effects of the dermal fillers immediately and increased effects over the course of the first 24–48 h. Follow-up care is at the discretion of the clinician, but patients should be uniformly counseled to seek follow-up care in the event of any delayed-onset complications, as explained in the following section. In general, any concerning erythema, reticulated patterns, blanching, lumping, or skin desquamation warrants the attention of the clinician.

## Complications and How to Avoid Complications

Soft tissue filler injections are second only to botulinum neurotoxin injections as the most popular medical cosmetic procedure performed in the United States [17]. These injection procedures are becoming increasingly more popular along with the demand for less invasive facial rejuvenation procedures. Patients, in general, want noticeable results with minimal downtime: filler injections provide both.

The overall safety profile of soft tissue filler injections is excellent; however, complications can occur. In general, complications are classified based on severity (major vs. minor) as well as time of onset (immediate, early (24–48 h), and delayed). Minor complications of facial filler injection associated with the injection site, itself, include pain, edema, and erythema [42]. These complications are typically transient and resolve within a week without sequelae [42].

At times, injections made too superficially may lead to unwanted lumps or palpable beads of filler within the skin that may persist for several months. These may warrant treatment with hyaluronidase and soft tissue massage to hasten resolution of palpable skin irregularities. Misplacement of soft tissue filler may also lead to a suboptimal or cosmetically deforming result, particularly when injecting beside a scarred area. Certain compressed scars may resist precise placement of filler, which may lead to dermal elevation beside instead of directly beneath the affected area.

Hypersensitivity reactions are possible with bovine collagen injection due to circulating antibodies. Contraindications to collagen therapy include patients with hypersensitivity to bovine products or beef allergy, patients on steroids or immunosuppressive medications, patients with a history of autoimmune disease, or pregnancy [19]. However, these reactions do not occur after injection with HA products or allogenic collagen [19]. In fact, after the introduction of a more highly purified product containing lower amounts of protein, the incidence of hypersensitivity reactions after HA injection decreased to 0.02 % [43].

Importantly, infection at soft tissue filler injection sites is often mistaken as an "allergic reaction" and treated as such without improvement. It has been proposed that low-grade bacterial infection may play a role in delayed-onset adverse reactions in patients mistaken as having "hypersensitivity" reactions to soft tissue fillers, and as such these patients should be treated promptly and aggressively with antibiotics [43]. Also important to keep in mind when evaluating patients with skin or soft tissue reactions is the longevity of soft tissue facial fillers. Although they are traditionally thought of as having temporary effects, Restylane has been reported to persist as long as 5 years after injection [21].

Rarely, reactivation of herpetic eruptions and localized bacterial infection may occur in susceptible patients [19]. These patients should be promptly and aggressively treated with antivirals and local wound care.

In contrast to minor skin edema or erythema following soft tissue filler injection, any immediate or early skin blanching, skin with a dusky or purple color, or skin with violaceous changes in a reticular pattern must be considered to be a manifestation of impending skin necrosis until proven otherwise [42]. Impending skin necrosis results from interruption of the vascular supply of the affected site and is a major complication of soft tissue filler injection. This complication has been reported in association with all types of filler, with an estimated incidence of 0.001 % for collagen and HA (Fig. 6.5) [42].

Impending necrosis occurs as a result of vascular injury—when filler is directly injected into the blood vessel supplying a particular skin territory or into an area adjacent to and resulting in compression of the affected facial vessel. Certain areas are at higher risk of skin necrosis than others. Glabellar necrosis has been reported more

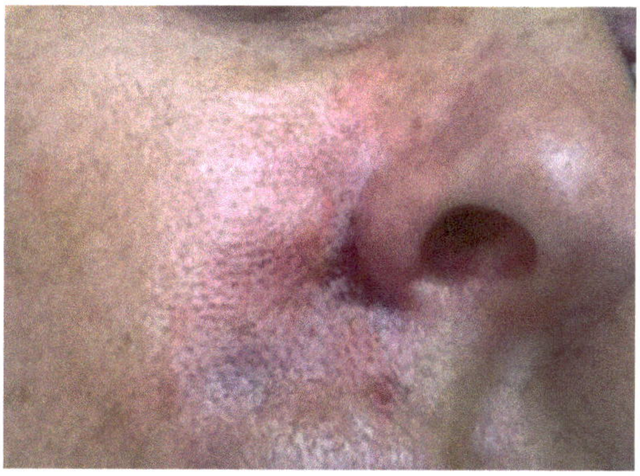

**Fig. 6.5** Impending necrosis 24 h following injection

**Table 6.1** Recognition and management of impending necrosis

| | |
|---|---|
| Presentation | Immediate or early blanching followed by a dusky or purple discoloration of the area |
| Treatment | Discontinue injection<br>Perform hyaluronidase skin testing<br>Inject 10–30 U of hyaluronidase per 2×2 cm area<br>Massage ½ in. of 2 % nitroglycerin paste into the area; apply warm compresses<br>Begin 325 mg ASA and an antacid regimen<br>Apply topical oxygen cosmeceutical therapy BID |
| Further management | Follow patient daily for further signs of occlusion/necrosis<br>Continue hyaluronidase and 2 % nitroglycerin paste daily as needed<br>Continue ASA, antacid, and topical oxygen therapy until wound has healed<br>If edema progresses, place on medrol dose pack<br>Consider hyperbaric oxygen for progressing necrosis resistant to the above-mentioned treatment options |

commonly than necrosis in the ala or nasolabial fold, likely due to a lack of collateral circulation in this area when branches of the microcirculation feeding off the supratrochlear artery are occluded [42]. Deeper injections are also more prone to this complication.

A protocol for impending skin necrosis (Table 6.1) published by Dayan et al includes immediately discontinuing the injection, followed by injecting 10–30 units of hyaluronidase (after hyaluronidase skin testing to assure no allergic reaction to the substance), applying 1/2 in. of 2 % nitroglycerin paste to the site, massaging the area with warm compresses, initiating aspirin (and antacid) therapy, applying topical oxygen (Dermacyte Oxygen Concentrate, Oxygen Biotherapeutics, Inc., Durham, NC), and following the patient daily until clinical improvement is achieved [42]. Although, today, higher doses of hyaluronidase are recommended. As much as 150 units per 2 $cm^2$ area of vascular compromise is not recommended.

Uncommonly but catastrophically, inadvertent intravascular injection of filler agents may lead to embolic events complicated by irreversible loss of vision or cerebrovascular injury [19]. In a large retrospective chart review, Park et al. reviewed the medical records of patients injected with cosmetic fillers into the glabellar or nasolabial regions over a 9-year period to highlight the incidence of retinal artery occlusion [45]. The mechanism of this adverse event is the retrograde propulsion of injected material into the ophthalmic or retinal arteries via the supratrochlear, angular, or dorsal nasal arteries during glabellar or nasolabial area injections, followed by arterial occlusion [45, 46]. They found twelve patients who had suffered filler injection-associated retinal artery occlusion (incidence: autologous fat>hyaluronic acid>collagen). Each patient experienced immediate and painful blindness following the injection; one case progressed to brain infarction; and all had poor visual prognoses. Any patient who experiences a decline in visual acuity or ocular pain after injection should be considered to have experienced this complication until proven otherwise. Immediate ophthalmologic evaluation and brain MRI are indicated. Theoretically, treatments should be aimed at rapidly reducing intraocular pressure in order to dislodge the embolus to a more downstream location, although no safe, feasible, and reliable treatment exists for iatrogenic retinal embolism [46].

Some measures may minimize the risk of iatrogenic ophthalmic artery embolism during cosmetic facial injections. Injection of a local vasoconstrictor should be used whenever possible. Aspiration prior to injection should be practiced to rule out intravascular placement of the needle or cannula. In theory, the smaller the needle, the better. However, it seems intuitive that smaller diameter cannulas can more easily penetrate a vessel. Therefore, larger cannulas, 25–27 gauge, are recommended by the author. Blunt, flexible needles and cannulas are preferred to their sharp counterparts. Importantly, the volume of filler injection should be limited (<0.1 mL per pass), the pace of the injection should be slow, and the pressure used to inject the substance should be low [46].

## Conclusion

Soft tissue filler augmentation of the periorbital regions is a valuable tool in the plastic surgeon's armamentarium. When performed correctly, periorbital rejuvenation pedestals the eyes and draws attention to this very expressive area and away from the lower third of the face that is most commonly associated with signs of aging.

## References


1. Hamel RF. Female subjective and pupillary reaction to nude male and female figures. J Psychol. 1974;87(2d Half):171–5.
2. Aboyoun DCD, James M. The Hess pupil dilation findings: sex or novelty. Soc Behav Pers. 1998;26:415–9.
3. Laeng B, Falkenberg L. Women's pupillary responses to sexually significant others during the hormonal cycle. Horm Behav. 2007;52(4):520–30.
4. Grammer K, Fink B, Moller AP, Thornhill R. Darwinian aesthetics: sexual selection and the biology of beauty. Biol Rev Camb Philos Soc. 2003;78(3):385–407.
5. Hickman L, Firestone AR, Beck FM, Speer S. Eye fixations when viewing faces. J Am Dent Assoc. 2010;141(1):40–6.
6. Hoehl S, Wiese L, Striano T. Young infants' neural processing of objects is affected by eye gaze direction and emotional expression. PLoS One. 2008;3(6):e2389.
7. Nguyen HT, Isaacowitz DM, Rubin PA. Age- and fatigue-related markers of human faces: an eye-tracking study. Ophthalmology. 2009;116(2):355–60.
8. Dayan SH, Arkins JP, Gal TJ. Blinded evaluation of the effects of hyaluronic acid filler injections on first impressions. Dermatol Surg. 2010;36 Suppl 3:1866–73.
9. Dayan SH, Lieberman ED, Thakkar NN, Larimer KA, Anstead A. Botulinum toxin a can positively impact first impression. Dermatol Surg. 2008;34 Suppl 1:S40–7.
10. Dayan SH, Arkins JP, Vaswani D, Christopher K. An open-label, prospective study to assess altering self-esteem following calcium hydroxylapatite injections. *Anglais*. In Peer-review. [AU6]
11. Rzany B, Cartier H, Kestemont P, et al. Full-face rejuvenation using a range of hyaluronic acid fillers: efficacy, safety, and patient satisfaction over 6 months. Dermatol Surg. 2012;38(7 Pt 2):1153–61.
12. Dayan SH, Arkins JP, Patel AB, Gal TJ. A double-blind, randomized, placebo-controlled health-outcomes survey of the effect of botulinum toxin type A injections on quality of life and self-esteem. Dermatol Surg. 2010;36:2088–97.
13. Flint PW, Haughey BH, Lund VJ, Niparko JK, Richardson MA. Cummings otolaryngology: head & neck surgery review. 5th ed. Philadelphia, PA: Elsevier; 2010.
14. Czogala J, Goniewicz ML, Czubek A, Golabek K, Sobczak A. Effect of tobacco smoking on skin and mucosa appearance, ageing and pathological conditions. Przegl Lek. 2008;65(10):732–6.
15. Horoszkiewicz-Hassan M. Influence of natural active compounds on the skin in tobacco smokers. Przegl Lek. 2009;66(10):882–4.
16. Jones D, Hill K. Criteria of facial attractiveness in five populations. Hum Nat. 1993;4(3):271–96.
17. Dayan SH, Arkins JP. The subliminal difference: a new treatment philosophy. J Drugs Dermatol. 2012;11(3):10–1.
18. Tan K, Oh S-R, Priel A, Korn B, Kikkawa D. Surgical anatomy of the forehead, eyelids, and midface for the aesthetic surgeon. In: Massry GG, Murphy MR, Azizzadeh B, editors. Master techniques in blepharoplasty and periorbital rejuvenation. New York: Springer; 2011. p. 11–24.
19. Rohrich RJ, Arbique GM, Wong C, Brown S, Pessa JE. The anatomy of suborbicularis fat: implications for periorbital rejuvenation. Plast Reconstr Surg. 2009;124(3):946–51.
20. American Society of Plastic Surgeons 2011 Plastic Surgery Statistics Report. ASPS National Clearinghouse of Plastic Surgery Procedural Statistics. 2012; http://www.plasticsurgery.org/Documents/news-resources/statistics/2011-statistics/2011_Stats_Full_Report.pdf. Accessed April 19, 2012.
21. Buckingham ED, Bader B, Smith SP. Autologous fat and fillers in periocular rejuvenation. Facial Plast Surg Clin North Am. 2010;18(3):385–98.
22. Yanoff M, Duker JS. Ophthalmology. St. Louis, MO: Elsevier; 2008.
23. The American Society of Aesthetic Plastic Surgery. 2010 Statistics from The American Society of Aesthetic Plastic Surgery. 2011; http://www.surgery.org/sites/default/files/Stats2010_1.pdf. Accessed April 26, 2011.
24. Dayan SH, Arkins JP, Somenek M. Restylane persisting in lower eyelids for 5 years. J Cosmet Dermatol. 2012;11(3):237–8.
25. Wang F, Garza LA, Kang S, et al. In vivo stimulation of de novo collagen production caused by cross-linked

hyaluronic acid dermal filler injections in photodamaged human skin. Arch Dermatol. 2007;143(2):155–63.
26. Narins RS, Brandt FS, Dayan SH, Hornfeldt CS. Persistence of nasolabial fold correction with a hyaluronic acid dermal filler with retreatment: results of an 18-month extension study. Dermatol Surg. 2011;37(5):644–50.
27. Carruthers J, Cohen SR, Joseph JH, Narins RS, Rubin M. The science and art of dermal fillers for soft-tissue augmentation. J Drugs Dermatol. 2009;8(4):335–50.
28. Kablik J, Monheit GD, Yu L, Chang G, Gershkovich J. Comparative physical properties of hyaluronic acid dermal fillers. Dermatol Surg. 2009;35:302–12.
29. Gold M. Aesthetic update: what's new in fillers in 2010? J Clin Aesthetic Dermatol. 2010;3(8):36–45.
30. Sundaram H, Voigts B, Beer K, Meland M. Comparison of the rheological properties of viscosity and elasticity in two categories of soft tissue fillers: calcium hydroxylapatite and hyaluronic acid. Dermatol Surg. 2010;36 Suppl 3:1859–65.
31. Lemperle G, Morhenn V, Charrier U. Human histology and persistence of various injectable filler substances for soft tissue augmentation. Aesthetic Plast Surg. 2003;27(5):354–66; discussion 367.
32. Hamilton DG, Gauthier N, Robertson BF. Late-onset, recurrent facial nodules associated with injection of poly-l-lactic acid. Dermatol Surg. 2008;34(1):123–6.
33. Mazzola RF, Cantarella G, Torretta S, Sbarbati A, Lazzari L, Pignataro L. Autologous fat injection to face and neck: from soft tissue augmentation to regenerative medicine. Acta Otorhinolaryngol Ital. 2011;31(2):59–69.
34. Dayan SH. What is beauty, and why do we care so much about it? Arch Facial Plast Surg. 2011;13(1):66–7.
35. Schiller D, Freeman JB, Mitchell JP, Uleman JS, Phelps EA. A neural mechanism of first impressions. Nat Neurosci. 2009;12(4):508–14.
36. Willis J, Todorov A. First impressions: making up your mind after a 100-ms exposure to a face. Psychol Sci. 2006;17(7):592–8.
37. Bar M, Neta M, Linz H. Very first impressions. Emotion. 2006;6(2):269–78.
38. Winston JS, O'Doherty J, Kilner JM, Perrett DI, Dolan RJ. Brain systems for assessing facial attractiveness. Neuropsychologia. 2007;45(1):195–206.
39. Richetin J, Croizet J-C, Huguet P. Facial make-up elicits positive attitudes at the implicit level: evidence from the implicit association test. Curr Res Soc Psychol. 2004;9(11):145–65.
40. Hickman L, Firestone AR, Beck FM, Speer S. Eye fixations when viewing faces. J Am Dent Assoc. 2010;141(1):40–6.
41. Cunningham MR, Roberts AR, Barbee AP, Druen PB, Wu C-H. Their ideas of beauty are, on the whole, the same as ours: consistency and variability in the cross-cultural perception of female physical attractiveness. J Pers Soc Psychol. 1995;68(2):261–79.
42. Grammer K, Fink B, Møller AP, Thornhill R. Darwinian aesthetics: sexual selection and the biology of beauty. Biol Rev Camb Philos Soc. 2003;78(3):385–407.
43. Studer LH, Aylwin AS, Reddon JR. Testosterone, sexual offense recidivism, and treatment effect among adult male sex offenders. Sex Abuse. 2005;17(2):171–81.
44. Dabbs JM, Jurkovic GJ, Frady RL. Salivary testosterone and cortisol among late adolescent male offenders. J Abnorm Child Psychol. 1991;19(4):469–78.
45. Park SW, Woo SJ, Park KH, Huh JW, Jung C, Kwon OK. Iatrogenic retinal artery occlusion caused by cosmetic facial filler injections. Am J Ophthalmol. 2012;154(4):653–62. e651.
46. Lazzeri D, Agostini T, Figus M, Nardi M, Pantaloni M, Lazzeri S. Blindness following cosmetic injections of the face. Plast Reconstr Surg. 2012;129(4):995–1012.

# Periorbital Fat Grafting: The 3D Lift

7

Mark Berman

The eyes are probably the most intimate aspect of anyone's appearance. As cosmetic and plastic surgeons, we have mainly focused on the vertical dimensions of the upper eyelid and aspects of redundant fat or skin in the lower eyelid. By now, it should be apparent that there is an important three-dimensional element to the periorbital area—something that has largely been neglected until recently. Now, we understand the importance of not just lifting the tissues upward or removing "unwanted" fat, but rather of lifting the skin in a specific anterior direction away from the underlying skeleton and soft tissue structures it covers [1].

While there is a time and place for traditional tissue excisional procedures, the importance of filling cannot be overemphasized. Today, a myriad of physicians and nurses are using a variety of filler agents ("liquid face lift") to try to improve youthful appearance without surgical incisions and excisions. The concept of fat grafting by injection is not new, but understanding why this material is superior to others when properly used and how it actually works are still considered emerging concepts.

As physicians we have the responsibility of first making a proper diagnosis prior to addressing a proposed therapy. Sadly, perhaps because the patient usually ends up looking better than prior to surgery, we have accepted traditional excisional procedures as the standard of care. Unfortunately, while many patients may be pleased with their surgical outcome, others often regret performing the operation because instead of "recapturing their youth" they removed "excess tissues" that resulted in a change in their eyelid appearance from what they had envisioned. Unless a youthful patient doesn't like their primary appearance, most aging patients would simply like to look like they used to. They tend to have a youthful vision of themselves within their mind and don't regularly accept the aging image seen in the mirror. Fundamentally, people want to look youthful as they used to appear. They don't usually want to look different and by all means, they don't want to look like they've had surgery.

Because we've misdiagnosed the causes for the appearance of aging, excisional treatments may make the patient look better by ridding them of unsightly rhytids, but it alone cannot restore their previous natural youthful image. Excisional procedures will positively affect the superior and posterior vectors, but generally, they decrease the anterior vector—just the opposite of what is normally required. To restore youthful appearance one must move the skin in a slight anterior position away from the skeleton, not closer to the skeletal structures [2–12] (Fig. 7.1).

Electronic supplementary material The online version of this chapter (doi:10.1007/978-1-4614-8388-5_7) contains supplementary material, which is available to authorized users.

M. Berman, M.D., F.A.C.S. (✉)
Facial Plastic Surgery, University of Southern California, Los Angeles, CA, USA
e-mail: markbermanmd@yahoo.com

S.A. Myint (ed.), *Nonsurgical Peri-orbital Rejuvenation*, DOI 10.1007/978-1-4614-8388-5_7,

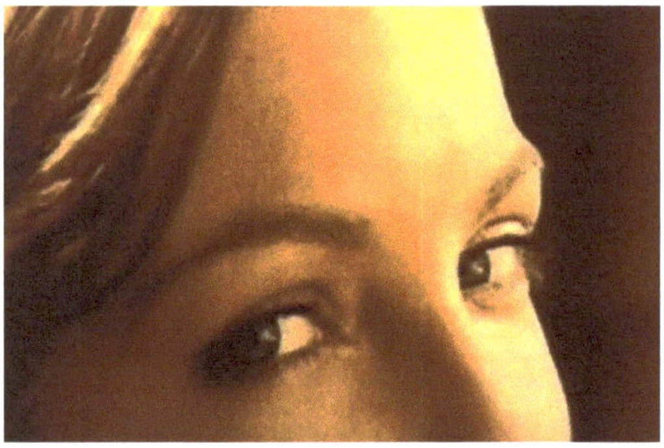

**Fig. 7.1** A youthful brow is contoured. The anterior vector or position of the brow needs to be understood and positioned in order to re-create an attractive eyelid

We have long assumed that our faces and periorbital area, in particular, are victims of age that degrades our skin and subcutaneous muscles to the point that gravitational forces can stretch and lengthen these elements. We now know that there are significant volume losses, particularly from subcutaneous fat, that are mostly responsible for this apparent downward descent of the tissues as well as the visualization of "pseudo-herniated fat pads." It's important to understand that fat cells have a finite length of survival (probably all cells do). Based on research by Yoshimura and others, it appears fat cells survive for 7–10 years. Once they succumb to death, neighboring stem cells are signaled to replace them. At some point, one must also run out of these regenerative cells. This is seen most notably on the face where subtle volume losses can effect millimeters of change that can significantly impact one's appearance. By understanding the process of fat cell death, depletion of regenerative replacement cells, and the necessity to restore the three-dimensional nature of the facial skin, one can see that fat, replete with regenerative (stem) cells, is the optimal physiologic choice for the most natural replacement tissue [13]. Of course, it requires a surgical procedure and generally some form of sedation to be best accomplished; however, because of the volume requirements and the long-lasting nature of the material, it remains ideal as a subcutaneous filler.

Many will argue that the hyaluronic acid fillers are superior because they are not long lasting and they can be reduced with hyaluronidase in the event of over corrections; however, one generally needs much more than a few cc's of solution and no face naturally contains hyaluronic acid. Likewise, this can be said for the other nonpermanent filler substances. And, while there are those that argue they prefer permanent implants or permanent fillers for long-lasting results, as long as the patient is alive, they will continue to metabolize fat and eventually the permanent materials will become apparent and they will require further camouflage—probably with fat grafting [14].

Arguably, many doctors are concerned about placing fat around the eyelid area because they fear it will leave disfiguring lumps and fail to correct the physical appearance as well as traditional excisional procedures. While one can easily find ways to disfigure a patient with fat, the list of complications that can occur with traditional procedures should provide some solace for one considering the procedure. Fundamentally, there are only two significant complications that could occur from fat grafting—a poor result or an infection.

A poor result is simply due to artistic ability or inability. Because we are literally sculpting the patient from the inside out, while we mark the patient prior to surgery as a guide to where volume is needed, we are dependent upon our visual senses to decide that the proper reshaping has been accomplished. So while there is some technical skill required and an understanding of where you must and must not place graft material, one is dependent upon their artistic judgment for optimal outcomes—something that concerns most physicians and surgeons. While most surgeons develop and subsequently possess good technical skills, far fewer are truly artistic.

It's probably better to under correct than try to over correct. Simple examples of problems occur from too much placement of fat, though, generally, most problems are simply related to not enough fat "taking" or the need for additional grafting. Patients should be advised to maintain a normal body weight. Significant increases in body weight could show up as significant changes in one's face. This is rare but I've seen it occur in a couple patients.

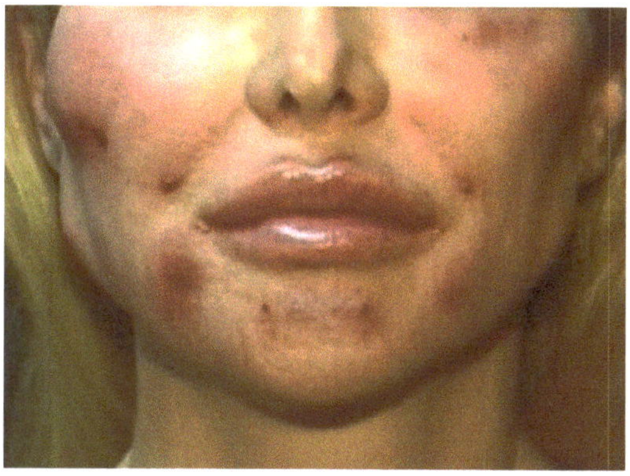

**Fig. 7.2** While rare, bacteria can be introduced into the graft site via dental infection or other blood-borne sources. Advise your patients to fix any dental problems prior to surgery

As for infection, it is largely avoidable. Since we are performing a sterile procedure with autologous materials, it's unlikely that we are providing a contaminant to the graft. However, we are causing trauma in multiple areas. This results in bleeding into the traumatized area. Of course, we've introduced a great culture medium (i.e., fat). So, from where does the bacteria come? I submit that one must be certain that your patient is free from any obvious source of blood-borne infection, particularly via the dental route. As such, I admonish all of my patients to care for any dental issues prior to surgery, not right after the operation. Any bacteria introduced into the blood stream can thus be introduced into the traumatized area and seed around the fat. If one picks up an atypical mycobacteria from the oral cavity or via dental intervention, this could lead to a very difficult infectious situation. Further, should a patient have a history of herpes or shingles in the area of injection, then prophylaxis with an anti-herpetic should be recommended and the patient advised of the possible risk of a "break-out" (Fig. 7.2).

Autologous fat transfer is not a matter of simply placing a layer of fat and hoping the body reconnects with the material. Thanks to the work of several plastic surgeons, we have a much better understanding for how this graft material actually works. Further, these principals have helped us to understand many concepts about adipose-derived stromal (stem) cells. Most body fat deposits are incredibly abundant with these regenerative or stem cells. The same hemopoietic stem cells found in bone marrow can be found in far greater abundance within fat tissue. Based on studies by Yoshimura and his group, we now understand that when you graft fat, you are actually doing a stem cell/fat graft. The fat cells suffer from hypoxia and as they die, they thus signal the stem cells to differentiate into supporting tissues, e.g., new fat cells and blood vessels, to connect and support the cells. Some of the fat cells survive. Some cells die and are eventually resorbed. It's a dynamic process.

## How I Do It

In general, most aging patients and even some younger ones, lack fat around the orbit and need to reposition their skin in a finite dimension away from the brow or cheek. The upper eyelid generally shows sagging of the brow secondary to volume loss, but it may present with deep hollowing, also secondary to volume loss. Often as periorbital and brow fat is lost, the appearance of bulges of intraorbital fat appear. This is generally explained to be pseudo-herniated fat, but this is simply a visualization of normal intraorbital contents made visible by the lack of fat lifting the skin away from these structures. Removing this fat (the generally accepted procedure) only serves to make the eyelids appear more hollow and affectively decompress (regardless to what extent) the intraorbital compartment. Decreasing fat within the eye socket simply allows the eye to start a retrograde descent into the orbit, something that really makes one look older.

Thus, for most upper lid changes associated with age, the basic plan is to restore the position of the brow. In the simplest situations, one only needs 1–3 cc of fat placed around the upper brow over the periosteal tissues and deep to the orbicularis oculi muscle of the upper eyelid. With losses of temporal fat, there is a lateral descent of the brow and this fat should likewise be replaced—typically over the superficial temporal fascia. And for more aggressive descent of the brow due to additional volume loss in the forehead, one must consider lifting the forehead anteriorly with placement of fat there as well. The skin over the forehead is too adherent to the frontalis muscle to be able to place fat in between the skin and the muscle without seeing lumps; therefore, it is safer to place fat deep to the frontalis muscle. Technically, one is placing the fat in a rather avascular plane, the galea aponeurosis, but due to the ability of the stromal cells to form blood vessels, it can actually survive.

In some cases, particularly older individuals, the upper eyelid skin may become so lax that a small excision of skin and/or a strip of muscle may be necessary. Of course, any pathology, such as true ptosis or other conditions, may need further operative attention or, depending upon your level of competency, referral to an ophthalmic plastic surgeon.

The lower lid generally presents with the appearance of increasing "bags" with advancing age. In some cases, there is increased hollowing under the lower lid, not infrequently due to iatrogenic removal of fat. In order to correct these defects, it's important to understand the basic cause. The bag does not appear because of increased fat volume in the orbit and pseudoherniation as we've generally been taught. While there may be circumstances where there is an actual increase in orbital volume resulting in additional fat bulging against the lower orbital septum, this is infrequent. In the extreme, one may see this with Grave's exophthalmos. In such cases, not only is the fat protruding, but because of the constriction of the orbital septum, the fat can only protrude so much and then the entire globe starts to protrude, thus causing the severe bulging appearance of the eyes familiar with this condition. Treatment of this condition requires removal of fat and often opening of the adjacent sinuses in order to decompress the orbit. Traditional blepharoplasty with fat removal likewise causes decompression of the orbit, although to a smaller degree that largely goes unnoticed, though not always by the patient.

Freeing the arcus marginalis and allowing lower orbital fat to slide inferiorly will often remove the demarcation of the lower lid bag or hollow. This can also be done in combination with fat grafting, but quite often just filling the cheek/lid tissues gets the same result without the additional surgery.

Patient selection criteria are fairly straightforward. Your patients generally are coming to you because they don't like the appearance of the area around their eyes. While this is most frequently seen with signs of aging, it's not unusual to see young people with bags or hollows that bother them as well.

A general history and physical exam will determine your patient's suitability for the potential surgical procedure. The procedure is most often done under intravenous sedation and local anesthesia.

For older individuals that want to look like they used to, ask them to bring a youthful photograph that they would like to resemble. Use it as a guide. Younger patients with other problems can bring photos of the kind of eyes they would like to have on their own face. This helps bridge any communication gaps. You may think you know exactly what would improve your patient's appearance and yet, be completely surprised by the youthful photo they'd like to duplicate. Their best image inside their head could be fairly different from what you might expect. It happens.

Preoperative photographs are essential. The key is to take them with consistent lighting from an overhead position in order to see all the necessary shadows. With direct flash lighting you can essentially wipe out the annoying shadows that the patient would like to eliminate. Direct flat lighting should be avoided.

Mark you patient in an upright position. Around the eyelids you may need to place fat into the forehead, brow, glabellar area, temporal area, and the cheek. I'll go over the proper placement in each of these areas. During the operation, you may prefer to keep your patient in a semi-seated position so you can more easily observe and judge the level of correction as you progress. In time, you may be comfortable with the patient in a supine/recumbent position, perhaps raising their head from time to time toward the end of the procedure.

The patient is further marked for the donor site that requires the initial liposuction. If the patient has a fat dysmorphia, then this is the ideal site. If there is no area where the shape can be improved, then you should find an area where fat removal will be least noticeable. This is often in the posterior hip area for most patients. In older women or postpartum women, the abdomen, though often replete in fat, may suffer from such poor skin tone that it can be very difficult to harvest fat and get a smooth result. This needs to be discussed with the patient ahead of time, of course. Finally, some patients are difficult to harvest fat without getting a defect in the area of removal. This needs to be discussed and might be a rate-limiting factor in proceeding with the operation. Nonetheless, a well-informed patient can responsibly make the decision in most cases [15].

Patients must also understand that they are likely to need a touch-up procedure. I remind all my patients that if "they're not willing to repeat the procedure, then don't do it at all." I charge a reduced fee for touch-ups, but that's up to you and you might want to consider it on a patient-to-patient basis depending upon the needs of the patient and your eventual experience. In the past (and probably currently), fat grafting not infrequently would receive negative comments from patients or doctors with little or no experience. It's not unusual for a patient to perceive a lack of improvement and comment that the procedure didn't work. Fat grafting always works. The problem is that there is variability from patient to patient regardless of your particular technique. Most likely, this is a function of stem cell population (concentration) within the fat graft and, to some extent, technique. There are other variables as well. Some surgeons strongly espouse the need to place fat into or around muscle tissue to enhance revascularization, but this isn't necessary. The face is very vascular, but more importantly, it's largely the regenerative cells within the graft that are responsible for angiogenesis and this can happen in areas of rather low vascularity. It should be obvious that you want your patient to be as healthy as possible, do light activities for at least the first week after the procedure, eat a healthy diet, and avoid anything that could be toxic to the new graft (e.g., smoking or any other potential irritant or infectious agent).

In the operating suite, the patient is placed in a supine position and your anesthetist can start an IV (or do it in the pre-op setting) and then position your patient supine or prone in order to harvest the fat. In the event that your patient must be pronated to harvest fat from the posterior hips, thighs, flanks, or back, then they can later be turned to a supine position using a simple "sheet" method. After the harvest, the patient's arms are carefully placed along their side. Another full sheet is then placed over the patient and grasped at the elbows (usually by the surgeon or strongest person) and at the knees by the surgical assistant or circulator. The anesthetist sole responsibility is to support the head. The patient can then be rotated (usually so the IV rotates superiorly) with veritable ease.

After years of trying a multitude of different techniques, I have been using a fairly simple and ingenious machine since 2008. Dr. Hee Young Lee developed the Lipokit (marketed in the USA by Palomar as the Adivive) and the associated syringes that make it an ideal fat processing system. With the patient under intravenous sedation, local anesthesia can be delivered either by tumescent injection using the Lipokit system or by simple injection using a 60 cc syringe via a spinal needle (22 g × 3½ in.). The entry port is initially injected with local via a 30 g needle. If using tumescent solution, we'll typically add 50 cc of 2 % lidocaine with epinephrine 1:100,000 and 10 cc of 8.4 % sodium bicarbonate into a 500 cc bag of normal saline. This gives a 0.2 % solution of lidocaine and for fat harvesting this is a very acceptable amount of lidocaine.

If using one or two syringes of local via a spinal needle, then a 0.5 % solution of lidocaine might be sufficient. Once the patient is sedated, a wheal is made with the local and a 30 g needle. If using the spinal needle technique, then the local is introduced directly below the skin to block the dermatome plexus of nerves that pass down through the skin to the fat. Tumescent anesthesia is effective, easier to do, and quicker, but it also adds a lot more solution to the harvest. Ultimately, when you are done with the harvest, you are going to centrifuge this material to separate the local, free fatty acids and condense the fat/stem cell population. You can probably get richer concentrations of fat without all of the tumescent and consequently save some money on syringes depending upon how much fat you need for a selective case. This will come with experience. The average patient needs around 45–60 cc of fat, so most often two 60 cc syringes will be needed for the harvest, but at times this could be much less or much more.

Once the patient has been properly anesthetized, then a sterile prep and drape is done. The Lipokit (Adivive) system is a completely closed system, so while it's recommended to use hat, mask, sterile gloves, and sterile drape, one does not need to be excessive in the process. Remember, at no time is the patient's fat being exposed to the atmosphere as it is always within a sterile syringe prior to being transferred into the recipient site.

A simple stab incision is made with a no. 11 blade or an awl depending upon your preference. Should you anticipate a lot of friction motion over the wound, you might want to use a plastic protective device. A 3.0 or 2.5 mm cannula connected to a Lipokit (Adivive) fat processing syringe is used. I'm not certain there is any benefit to the type of cannula you use or the aperture size of the holes in it, though others have argued that smaller holes help break up the cells into smaller and more accessible particles. Recent studies have suggested it doesn't matter whether you centrifuge the cells or wash them in a simple strainer. I've tried nearly all techniques and have settled on this one over the last several years for a variety of reasons. First, it was simple. I got it right the first time I tried it. Next, it was completely enclosed and eliminated handling as a possible source of contamination. Further, my surgical tech loved that there was no mess as she usually had associated with processing fat. The centrifuged fat is actually compressed by a special weighted piston so that the concentration of stem cells within the fat is maximized for that patient. This should further improve the results of the procedure.

Once the cannula is introduced, the fat can be harvested. It's important to understand, regardless of which equipment is used with the syringe, that the harvest process is the same technique as any syringe liposuction. If one uses the machine with its continuous aspirator, they need to understand that the suction is being provided to the weighted piston and that the actual suction for the fat harvest is from the area between the cannula and the piston. Thus, if the cannula tip should be pulled back so that air can be encountered, then the suction will be lost and the dead space must be expelled prior to reinserting the cannula and starting the suction process again.

Once the harvest process is complete, the syringe or syringes (up to four) are placed in the centrifuge. The centrifuge is set at 2,800 RPM and spun for 3 min. Initially, I've used the parameters of 4,000 RPM for 8 min as this further increases concentration of the fat and stem cells. There's concern that it also decreases cell viability so the lower speed and time have been used largely based upon my communications with Dr. Yoshimura and Dr. Lee. It might be reasonable to use the higher parameters in someone that has a lot of fat so you could try to maximize stem cell concentration at the sake of viability. Since 2010, I've been using the lower parameters with fairly good (consistent) results.

Prior to placing the syringes in the centrifuge, it's important to loosen the screw on the top of the weighted piston. Within the piston is a 100 μm filter. By loosening the screw, the piston can force itself upon the fat and yet allow free fatty acids from broken or fragile cells to escape through the filter for eventual easy disposal.

While the fat is being prepared in the centrifuge, you can start anesthetizing the face with local anesthesia. For periorbital grafting, I use lidocaine 1 % with epinephrine 1:100,000 and 1 cc of 8.4 % sodium bicarbonate per 10 cc syringe. I'll inject with a 27 g needle starting at the supraorbital nerve and then infiltrating a small amount along the brow. If forehead grafting is anticipated, I'll deliver local deep to the frontalis. It can be delivered in the area of the glabella just under the skin. In the lateral brow, a layer of local can be infiltrated into the temporal area well into the hairline. In the cheek, it is delivered to the infraorbital foramen and then infiltrated down to the bone and just under the skin of the entire cheek. This can be done from the middle of the cheek but also should include the corner of the mouth as that will most often be the preferred entry site for the eventual graft.

After each area is infiltrated, it is advised that you stop or an assistant hold pressure over the area for at least 1 min. This will significantly help limit ecchymosis that largely occurs from the needle injury to small vessels that then bleed prior to coagulating. Pressure on these tiny puncture wounds should help reduce some of the inevitable bruising. Prolonged bruising seems to be more bothersome to patients than the significant swelling they will complain about the first 2 days in particular. Most edema subsides by the end of a week. Ecchymosis, in severe cases, can lasts for 3 or more weeks. Compression after injection will significantly reduce this time.

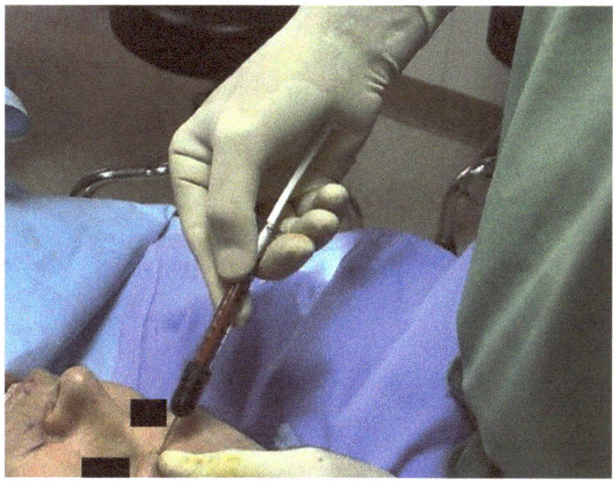

**Fig. 7.3** Precise control is easier to maintain by injecting tiny amounts with the syringe plunger held against the back of the palm

An 18 g needle is used to make an entry wound for blunt cannula introduction. Bilaterally, entry wounds are made at the medial brow, lateral brow, and corner of the mouth. Fat is transferred to 1 cc syringes and then the 1.4 mm blunt cannula is applied. I usually begin at the medial brow area and inject the upper eyelid first. The syringe should be held so that the plunger lies in the palm of your hand and pressure to the plunger can be administered very precisely in very small increments. Typically, the cannula is advanced over the inferior portion of the brow over the periosteum, deep to the orbicularis oculi, and fat is carefully infiltrated while withdrawing the cannula. Fat can be introduced all the way down to the upper lid sulcus and used to fill out sagging or hollow upper lids. It can be delivered in tiny amounts so as to smoothly as possible fill out the "deflated" brow and upper lid complex. Fat can also be introduced above the brow and well into the forehead, taking care to stay deep to the frontalis muscle in order to avoid lumping surely to occur above the frontalis muscle. In the glabellar area, one can inject fat more superficially, just under the skin and over the corrugator muscles. By filling in the forehead, this not only achieves a rounder more youthful appearance, it helps to elevate the brow as well (Fig. 7.3).

Through the lateral brow entry point, the cannula is advanced just over the temporalis muscle and carefully fanned out around the temporalis, often going well into the hairline. The fat must be carefully placed in fine amounts so that it spreads over the temporalis smoothly without lumps.

Once the upper face has been completed, attention is turned to the lower lid and cheek. Via the corner of the mouth entry wound, the cannula is advanced deep over the periosteum. Ideally, one can help raise the corner of the mouth with adequate fat grafting below the zygomaticus major. After layering fat deep to the facial muscles, it is then layered in a more superficial plane. Prior to surgery the areas are mapped and marked on the patient's face. In general, one wants to tent the skin away from the skeleton with the cheek apex being more prominent just below the orbital foramen. Use the old photos as a guide. The fat is then tapered to raise this area and can even be placed over the orbital septal fat but must remain deep to the orbicularis oculi muscle. Anything above the muscle will leave lumps under the very thin skin. The fill is continued laterally to the extent that the patient needs or wants it. Some patients want slightly exaggerated cheekbones, while most want the cheeks to blend into the lower face without too much lower cheek hollowing. Again, review the patient's favorite photos to determine their preferences. By lifting the skin away from the face in an anterior direction, you will thus "tent" the skin away from the skeleton so that you will no longer see the underlying skeletal structures. It's essential to lift the skin away

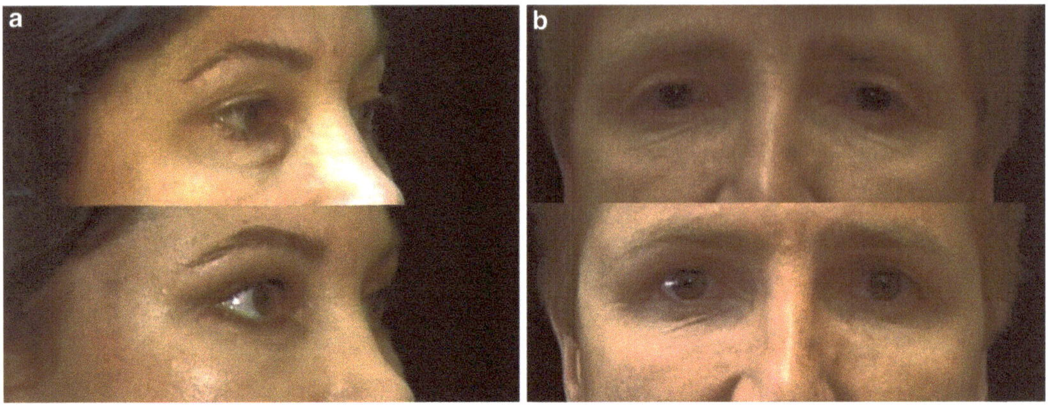


**Fig. 7.4** (**a**) Without excision of skin, contours are restored with fat grafting in a three-dimensional manner. (**b**) Redundant tissues and lower lid bags or hollows are filled to lift skin away from the skeleton and restore more youthful contours without excision. In some cases, a minor excision of skin can be complimentary

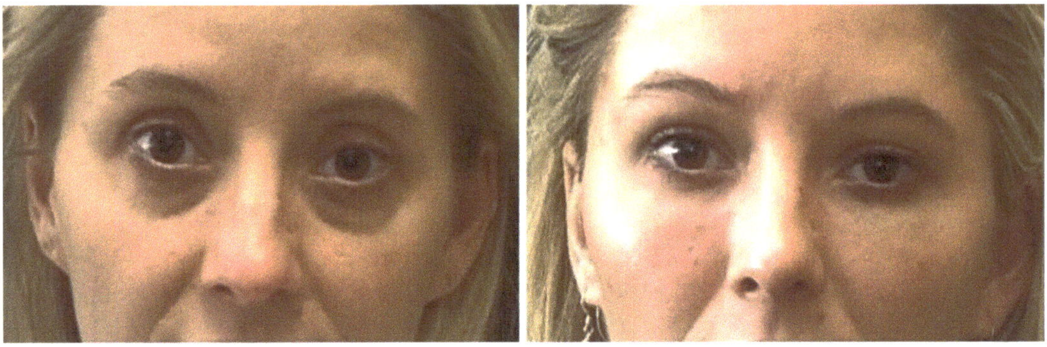

**Fig. 7.5** Congenital hollowing occurs and is corrected by filling in areas around the orbit and cheek to provide and more pleasant contour

from the underlying tissues in this "global" manner and not try to simply fill in perceived defects. Even patients with very significant "lower lid bags" can have the appearance of the bag removed by simply filling in the cheek skin and not excising the fat (Figs. 7.3, 7.4, 7.5, 7.6, and 7.7).

Generally, wherever you inject the fat, that's where it will remain. In the event that you inject too much into one area, you can either try to aspirate it right away or even apply some pressure to try to disperse it. Grafting should be done as carefully as possible, of course, but interestingly, we've observed that it can be fairly forgiving. Over time, it can even improve the quality of the underlying tissues—possibly due to the effects of the abundant mesenchymal stem cells. It's reasonable, therefore, to refrain from overcorrecting as it's easier to add more volume than to remove it. While it's highly unusual, it is possible for your patient to gain excessive weight and see their facial fat swell dramatically. Remind them to try to keep their weight stable. On the reverse side, patients that lose substantial weight after fat grafting will likely lose some volume in their face too—just as they would under normal circumstances.

Subsequent to the procedure your patient should be advised to have light activity for the next week. They should try to sleep with their head elevated on a few pillows to help with the swelling. The first 2 days after the operation can exhibit a lot of edema. Patients need to be reassured that while they may look terrible for a few days, it is temporary and if they looked good in the operating room, it is impossible for you to create more volume than what you added during surgery and they are simply seeing edema. A lot

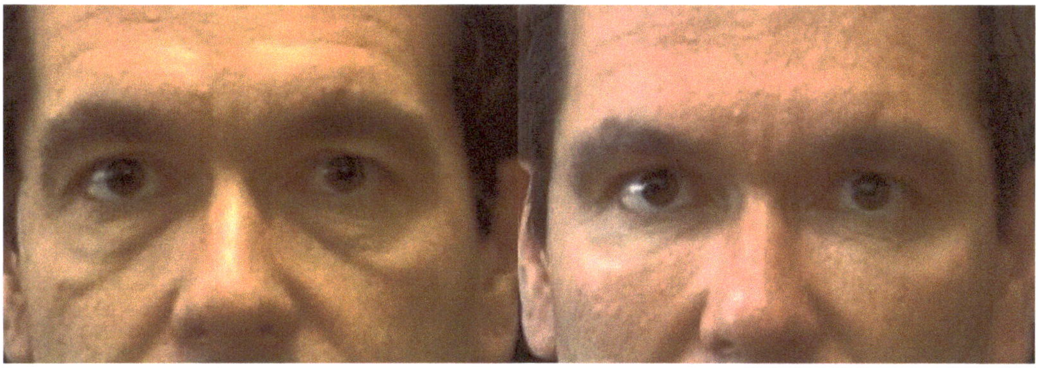

**Fig. 7.6** Sagging around the periorbital region often includes lines formed by a prominent malar ligament. When the skin is positioned away from the skeleton and contours are repositioned, then this problem is corrected in a natural manner

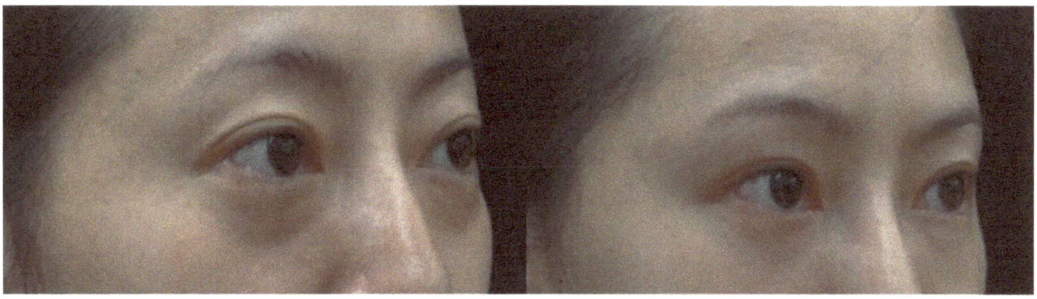

**Fig. 7.7** Subtle contour changes around the periorbital area with fat grafting can restore more youthful contours. The changes may be subtle but are necessary to avoid iatrogenic problems associated with excisional procedures

of patients think it's a good idea to consume large quantities of water; however, this may further aggravate their edema and I advise them to hydrate normally and avoid excessive water consumption. On the same token, I recommend they have a normal diet and don't use the time to try to restrict their calories. It's quite likely that it doesn't matter what we request of our patients, short of vigorous exercise, as the real determinant of success is dependent on the quality of the graft and its concentration of stem cells.

## References


1. Berman M. The aging face: a different perspective on pathology and treatment. Am J Cosmetic Surg. 1998;15(2):167–72.
2. Millard DR, Yuan RTW, Devine JW. Challenge to the undefeated nasolabial folds. Plast Reconstr Surg. 1987;80(1):37–46.
3. Riefkohl R. The nasolabial fold lift. Ann Plast Surg. 1985;15(1):1–6.
4. Yousif NJ, Gousain A, Matlojub HS, et al. The nasolabial fold: an anatomic and histologic reappraisal. Plast Reconstr Surg. 1994;93(1):60–8.
5. Robbins LB, Brothers DB, Marshall DM. Anterior SMAS plication for the treatment of prominent nasomandibular folds and restoration of normal cheek contour. Plast Reconstr Surg. 1995;96(6): 1279–87.
6. Knize DM. An anatomically based study of the mechanism of eyebrow ptosis. Plast Reconstr Surg. 1996;97(7):1321–42.
7. De la Plaza R, de la Cruz L. A new concept in blepharoplasty. Aesthetic Plast Surg. 1996;20:221–33.
8. De la Plaza R, de la Cruz L. Can some facial rejuvenation techniques cause iatrogenia? Aesthetic Plast Surg. 1994;18:205–9.
9. Gosain AK, Amarant MTJ, Hyde JS, Yousif NJ. A dynamic analysis of changes in the nasolabial fold using magnetic resonance imaging: implication for facial rejuvenation and facial animation surgery. Plast Reconstr Surg. 1996;98(4):622–36.
10. Stuzin JM, Wagstrom L, Kawamoto HK, Baker TJ, Wolfe SA. The anatomy and clinical application of the buccal fat pad. Plast Reconstr Surg. 1990;85(1): 29–37.

11. Paul MD. Subperiosteal transblepharoplasty forehead lift. Aesthetic Plast Surg. 1996;20:129–34.
12. Freund RM, Nolan WB. Correlation between brow lift outcomes and aesthetic ideals for eyebrow height and shape in females. Plast Reconstr Surg. 1996;97(7):1343–8.
13. Yoshimura K, Eto H, Harunosuke K, Kentaro D, Noriyuki A. In vivo manipulation of stem cells for adipose tissue repair/reconstruction. Regen Med. 2011;6(6 Suppl):33–41.
14. Coleman SR. Structural fat grafting. St. Louis, MO: Quality Medical; 2004.
15. Rohrich RJ, Sorokin ES, Brown SA. In search of improved fat transfer viability: a quantitative analysis of the role of centrifugation and harvest site. Plast Reconstr Surg. 2004;113(1):391–5.

# Erratum

## Nonsurgical Peri-orbital Rejuvenation

Shoib A. Myint

S.A. Myint (ed.), *Nonsurgical Peri-orbital Rejuvenation*, DOI 10.1007/978-1-4614-8388-5,


---

**DOI 10.1007/978-1-4614-8388-5_8**

**The order of authors on Chapter 5 as follows.**

Daniel I. Schlessinger
Northwestern University School of Medicine

Joel Schlessinger, MD, FAAD, FAACS
Director, Advanced Skin Research Center, Omaha, NE

Heidi A Waldorf, MD
Director, Laser & Cosmetic Dermatology
Mount Sinai Medical Center, and
Associate Clinical Professor
Icahn School of Medicine
New York, NY

Waldorf Dermatology & Laser Associates, PC
Nanuet, NY

---

The online version of the original book can be found at
http://dx.doi.org/10.1007/978-1-4614-8388-5

---

# Index



S.A. Myint (ed.), *Nonsurgical Peri-orbital Rejuvenation*, DOI 10.1007/978-1-4614-8388-5,

FSC
www.fsc.org
MIX
Papier | Fördert
gute Waldnutzung
FSC® C083411

Kolibri 360 GmbH
Ferdinand-Jühlke-Straße 7
99095 Erfurt, Deutschland
produktsicherheit@kolibri360.de